# And for a Moment Everything Seemed Fine

## Paul Fearne

**chipmunkapublishing**
the mental health publisher

All rights reserved, no part of this publication may be reproduced by any means, electronic, mechanical photocopying, documentary, film or in any other format without prior written permission of the publisher.

>Published by
>Chipmunkapublishing
>United Kingdom

**http://www.chipmunkapublishing.com**

Copyright © Paul Fearne 2025

ISBN    9781783827275

This book is written in poetic prose.

I have left a number of errors in this work to give it a fragmented feel.

This book is a treatise on suffering. It is the contention of this book that we can do things with our suffering to improve the quality of our lives. As individuals, when we encounter suffering, this book argues, our consciousness gets heightened, and we are able to direct this reflex towards things we want or need, thereby improving our lives. Our suffering leads to our mind manifesting the conditions of the possibility of improvement. I believe it is an evolutionary capacity. One grown out of repeated encounters human beings have had with suffering.

The manifestation we are here talking of can lead to a whole range of things we are interested in becoming realities – work, leisure, friends, partners, even more. All by confronting suffering front on and allowing our consciousness to heighten.

One can see this reflex at work in the history of poetry. People encountering great suffering, and direct that suffering towards their poetry. Why did William Blake produce drawings for the Book of Job? Because of his suffering of course.

I can think also of Vincent Van Gogh, who directed his suffering towards his art, thereby improving that aspect of his life.

Aside from giving the book a fragmental feel (which is important) the errors left in this book are a store of small sufferings ready for the reader to use for the purposes of improving their lives.

What will you do with your suffering?

(Just before we begin, a definitional point. I have used the term 'vicissitude' as a synonym for suffering in an idiosyncratic fashion. The 'variation of fortune' of the standard definition can, I believe, encompass suffering when experienced in the world.)

There – in the trees, the past has manifest. There is now something we should do, more than ever. Is this in the rule book? Is this where we look? Sounds of glass on glass. Tempest on tempest. This is what is said. We will fight the fight.

I must remember what it is I must say. To forget is to rub shoulders with the residue of life. There is something in me that harbours the unknown.
There is something in me that betokens the night. But what of the seam of the world?

And now, like a force that has no tide. Like a belief that heralds nothing but the sand we walk on. I am one to wind it through. I am one to see the lectern trolley itself into new main attempts. There is a tendency here to walk the mile we are set.

## And for a Moment Everything Seemed Fine

Do not winnow, it does not suit. Have the wind at our backs, and forages in the tendency of things. There comes a bliss, that has not so much as a righting of the ship. I will lunge forward and find something that is quite special – Yes.

Off we go – into southern and inexplicable climbs. What is this we seek? What is this we know of? Come, and build a fence around the world. We will not levy a fee for what are works of amazing ingenuity. Come now, find a way.

And then, like the powder in the keg, of we smart, to art and all that remains. Come and be a rounded figure in place full of rest. There is now something more we must do. And that is keep walking, despite the rain and its insistence. Yes, of course.

And then, compunction, and stated relief. I know of no other thing, no other thing that heralds daylight. Be the trapeze, and I will be your suffering. Come now, there is a gust of wind. I know how to be taught, in skills and language other than this.

And now, with a solemnity aging like fire, that says to the mass – repute or fail – there is here a weathering blast. Do not sense the age, feathers widow, and the sustenance that keeps us aloft wrangles in time, and out. Fever in lock.

And with, the holding of the balustrade, we recognise what it is that keeps us going. It is our heightening of consciousness, that does not linger, but rains in dimensions of levity. Moisten the bridges – hardship comes only to that which launches.

But what of this? What of the dancing in times of the lute? What of this entanglement that dreads the shadow of delay? We have what we need. We have all that we need. But what is left of us, we cannot tell. But we will bend in a wind that treasures.

What do we need – need from here? We need hope, hope in a future that has no parallel. Look there is suffering, let us take it! And use its effect upon us to gather in hope. That is our lot – we can do nothing but succeed.

A cloud. Rain. Misapprehension, a gathering to see things clearly. I will not send the chance to look again back to its encumbered land. Be brief, the stars will come. Be brief, and all that you surmise will come to pass. That is it.

## And for a Moment Everything Seemed Fine

Rocking the steel of it, until its strength shows no demise. There is suffering here – a suffering we have not seen in a quince. Formidable, and without science. Consecrate the nerve endings, and what you find will not wilt.

Holding on, and then whispering to the day. Lovely it is to flourish. Have time, and all that will be will be. Blistering for the density of it. Seeing things float, and having them wander. I will never believe in the wilderness of things. There, I have said it.

What do we do when the pain of it rises? We let it burrow in deep, and let our heart and mind soar. Let it change our life, so that we have what we need and want. Cautious now, the seeing we do will not change – not now at least.

Coming in close, we fire ourselves again, and know that the preamble of things has a heart just like us. I find the necessity of it all blinding. Give roughness to the dawn and what will come will be a litter of correspondences that dreams the dream.

Belief – it is a wonderful thing. It steels us, and carries us, and has as the bark of it a merriment that cannot be shaped to anything other than milk. I will cage the sun, and have it duly revoked, and then like a rapscallion dirge, repeat, and deliver.

Come now, we have not the sound of it to make us laugh. What is this we write? Is it sand on sand, water on water? Hedge on hedge? I will glean a sufficient condition, and then have what is left a solemn bath to wash away the tangles.


And then, like a tail in a nighttime cry, we hear ourselves relinquish the tethers that have held us, and then find them folded in the way of all things. Do not cry the cry yourself – let the world besiege what it is we most desire. Then, and only then.


And now, like destiny in the arc of it, we catch what it is that holds us back. And then, like a culinary port of call, we sense more than has ever been sensed. I have here something of the match and the kindling. There is now a fist to dry.


Like a ghost – in-between the covers of a worn-out life. There are things that move us, and things that herald day. We have a grand delectation. And here we whisper. Joy to things that bring. Joy to those who saunter. We will not faint.


If one thing disappears from our world – let the suffering become deep. And here there will be a change – maybe an inclusion. Our senses heightened, and simply we manifest what is needed. There is no auction about it.

The sea – I hear it. And then, like a time to reverberate – we sense also that leisure can come of its own accord. A distress never comes too soon. There is a witness to the daylight, that has as its edict more than we have encountered before.

What do you say? What speech do you use? The speech of the horizon? Or the speech of the motherland? Do not encounter what we say is not real. And here the distance that we have finally traversed will floor the world.

I see things differently now. There is less of this, but more of that. And then, like a touchstone that has no sight, but a hearing of all the realm, we linger – to say the least. I will corner you, and know the time to be set. Good.

What is this thing we seek? What can only be engraved in stone. There is a message from the beyond. What does it say? We suffer, but we redirect it. This much is what we can do. I will never lose hope. For this reason.

An arch way through and into the snow. I have heard it said, trunks of beating hearts will shiver, and then release. What can be said, has already been said. What is now, is now past. What was then is now gone. Do not despise.

Happenstance, and ranging through. What the eyes never see. What is most at odds. Climbing to get a better look. I will not hurry, this time, for anything or anyone. There is purpose here like nothing gone before. Impossible.

I will sense a new place. It is where suffering has no hold. It is where the vultures of today cannot gather. I will try my best, until something moves the path. Come now, visions do not pretend. I am there now, where the august and the strange begin.

Do we facilitate change, or does change facilitate us? There is a soaking that underlies the beauty of it all. I will see this thing above and below, and know that the heart is here for respite, and the chiselling of worn-down rock always works.

There is here and now a movement through far away places that has as its guiding scope more than measures in luxurious charm. I will hold myself the wanting and the day. And here, where the solemn and the cloudy move in equal path – a treasure.

Mischief – thine eyes! I will have something more to say. Come suffering, we will not let you pass. We will keep you until the rounds of this to that never fail us. I have seen more than is lightning. I have seen less than is fact. We will suffice.


A drum beat in the morning, soaring, and never letting go. I am one to wonder. I am one to scrawl in times of joy. I have in my bag all that has been and gone. There is a loneliness that can only be dispelled by one thing – the heart.


Have no fear, my whistling doesn't break the day, but holds itself in the motion and the benefit of all those that have started the chase. I love this time, when all is crisp, and the density of togetherness can only change what is ripe.


Dreaming – but of what? Lascivious, but for whom? We drag closer, and know that time will not stand still. Be the might, and your sword will conquer night. Be the victory, and the sense you have will guide you. Verily, and without danger


But we must continue. Do not let your suffering overpower you – but let it fill you. And this is the catalyst for change. Let your life improve and prosper. Do not be negligent in your duty. Things will come, and come they will. Indeed.


The time it takes. The weather – all around. Misgivings, and all that can cast a shadow. I will send things skyward, and know them to be the treasure they are. Foxing, and belligerent. In time to guess. I will come.


Cautious, with a sense of ruin. This is like nothing else, and nothing left. I hear you call, but do not respond. I hear your name, and it triggers something deep within. Do not catch the rhythm, it leads us astray. I have felt much – let us begin.


And now, like landfall, we find release. What comes in tune to a vibrant uncertainty. We live for this, and then for naught. I hear your voice, and send you salutations. What is this – what can be in times of gracious applause. There will be more to come.


Finding solace, in amongst the suffering. This is key. And then a witch, with all the trappings. I like what it is that we see. I like what it is that we turn for. I am certain, certain of this. I will conquer like none have. And here we must stay. Once again.


Following the lead – there is time. Following what we need – do not wish. There is a foundling in the midst. We will venture, and then swerve. Come now, oftentimes we will sing. And then, like trees in the light – we will cast a glow, and never fall.


I see myself in your reflection. I see what it is I have lost. But then, what is worth fighting for?

## And for a Moment Everything Seemed Fine

What stems from the ground, and silos up to top most care. I have found the motion – it is here. I have found the momentum - it comes in grains.


Is there more to it than this? All you do is let suffering rub up against you, and then let it fall. All you need is a template to begin – what will your suffering be for? And watch it make the improvement. It is not hard. It works for poets and artists.


What will the sands of togetherness bring? What has the twilight got to offer? I will see fate in the palm of all hands. And here, where the milk and honey of a generation comes to a standstill, I see the mischief of a side glimpsed world come together.


And now, without the furthest need, we come again to settle old scores. It is here where the mansion of our dreams laughs the loudest. I cannot see things as they were, but that doesn't matter – I will see anyway. Come and be torn.


Solid, and without the match to accompany all aspects of the dawn. I see what is now missing. It is me in pieces of rebellious tape. I see this not as an offering, but rather as a chance at greater things. We will never stop, for all things.

I see clearly now – it is as if the solstice has
caught itself on the feelings of all those who do not
feel. Come and be a wanderer in dead of night.
Come and silence the sound of the horizon at first
light. I will catch more than I can. I will not cease.


Flying and being entertained, I wish this were what
we had to believe in. But more of this in due
course. I have never been more in tune with
things. Come now, do not force yourself. Do not
water the mile. It comes to stay close.


Listening to the sound of the rain. It comes, and
then suddenly disappears. I wish for something
else, but the time it takes does not permit. I will
launch myself into nothingness, and have as an
anchor the air. This much will hold.


Can we call suffering for what it is? Can we use it
to defy what is next? And then, like a lingering
heart, we find ourselves anew. Just as a chasm in
waiting. Just as noise we wish to hear. I am one to
seek something new. And then? Who knows.


The castle remains. It has stood the test of things,
and knows how to live. I cannot remember the
time of my birth, only that which surrounds it. But
then, the tempest only shouts our name once, and
then retreats until the next aversion.

Liking what we see, there is a place that harbours no noise, nor no sense of pride. I gather myself for one last chance at togetherness, but that has as its fold the veerings of the wild and the life. Do not dispense with the ancient memory.


Gaining in speed, the vociferous and short meander forward, and know that the boisterous will commence without hesitation. I am one never to see things afresh. And here, like a garb in tandem, we whistle, and know things to be great.


And then, like tender hooks, we silence our greatest mystery. And like a river that does not flow, we see ourselves in the rain, and know that the herald will not pass. I see things that little bit clearer, and believe once again that things will be okay.


I have seen the test of it – and am not afraid. There is a whim about it that gathers strength. I have one feeling about this, and one feeling only – it will happen, and in time, we will see if that judgement stands. We will see.


Watching through the mist, we see ourselves wander. And then, like a window that looks out onto the sea – emotion, and the semblance of calm. I see you. I see you sitting there, and know you to be one to swim the mile. Let us relay.

Suffering – heightening – improvements – start again. Watch as we transform our world, from start to finish. Watch as things come together. Watch as the storm subsides. Forming an opinion, we no longer squirm.

Mixing things together, to make them smoother. I have often said that things are hard enough, why bond them stronger. And then, like wafer to behold, we settle in, and see the passage of it to be a wonder. I will never give in.

There was once a trial of hearts, that didn't feel itself portrayed in silk. I love this most dearly. Come now, do not be one to shirk – shirk the responsibility of an age. There is now something more to see, and I will see it, see it through.

Bringing on the wagon, we sit, and be still with life at our backs. Do not come most gently, we are full of arrows, and drive and wanderlust. I feel the morning quicken, as the pace of things enlivens. We must always be at one with what is most dear.

And then, like a cold mint at the station, there comes a cry that doesn't cease, and here, in the middle of it, the sound of something unknown. But that is what we thought – could it be different? I shed a tear for the dawn. There, I said it.

## And for a Moment Everything Seemed Fine

Bringing the night sky, we harbour what is most at stake. And what is this – it is love, and all that can fit inside it. I laugh, and see the plain diminish by halves. I feel what is closest to us, and that is something to applaud. And then like steel, we continue.


Hanging on, feeling like the road is going straight. There is never enough wood to carry us. There is never enough weather to find in check. I will lie still. I will give what we need to the dawn. And here, where chances are relished, a spring to tide.


What happens? A piece of suffering emerges. Embrace it, feel it, sense its strength. And then, through a natural reflex, transform it into something you need, or want. There is no going back. Once the result is seen, it becomes addictive.


I have heard it said, that the dice do not roll straight. But that is what we have come to see. I will linger, and watch as the time of it commences. But what of this, our lives? There is no cost – nothing to barter – Only what is fresh.


A string, and what the daylight has to give. I am fond of saying something picturesque, and then leaving it to dry. What of the sand, as it rolls on harbours indiscreet? I am one to see things again.

Much of it is like the rest. Much of it contains nothing we cannot see. I love this part, but what of the next? We will see it ballooning in motion to the clouds. There is like something we have never seen before. That will help.


A certain tally shows the way. In it, an adumbration of cards. Do not swell, it will not appeal. Come and be a quarter master in a realm of the indifferent. You are here to choose. And with that aligned with the merriment of things – again.


Now, like a whistling that has no sound, there is much to do, and much that we can say has been done. I have reached that point where laughter reigns, and the sweetness of it curtails. There can only be one thing to do – and that is begin.


What do we stand for? What is it that we bleed? I have known nothing other than this. I have known nothing other than the sky at dusk. I wish for you, as others do. I wish for farthings and treasures sent. There will be time – always.


I feel like the rock on Gibraltar stands – there is a mischief here, like the feeling we once had that the tempest will only opine. Come now, altered

## And for a Moment Everything Seemed Fine

mist – you are what is in turn believed in. I will not tarry, I can only see what is near.


Suffering, we encounter it, and let it go. It comes back at pace, but we let it go again, and then it is transformed, transformed into something else – improvements for us, and our lot is risen. There is nothing else to it.


And then like a woollen shawl, we cope. But where is the sound of longing, and where does it come from? I see no time to delay. We give ourselves all we can. And it is here we flourish, flourish like never before. We will never be tempered.


A joust, of this place to the next. I hear your sand – it is like a piece of cloth, ready to polish. And then like a runaway there comes a distant exposure, one that lingers it the midst of things. Do not court the time – it has its own juncture.


Warbling, and with an ease that surprises, there emerges a saying, in style and grace. What is it doing here? What is its purpose? Why can it not fly, but run like the distance? A belief comes next, and all that will follow.


Never caught in the crossfire, we tell ourselves of wondering missions, and larks in spaces of night.

Do not give credence to the shore – it only holds back beauty. And then, without recoil, there is a languishing in the sense of this to that. Yes.


Tethered – but tethered to what? Life, and all of its accoutrements. Be dazzling, and be all out. There is now a piece of land that thrives. It registers nothing, but has as its guide all the will of the world. I will nestle up close, and never come back down.


A pinch of pain – then look inside – what do we see? Something quite amazing. A glimpse of a heightened consciousness. It transforms all it encounters, and knows itself to be something untold – until now.


Verisimilitude, and what we feel. I have come to guard the weather – guard it from intensity. I have come, come to be something more. Do not rain on shores unblemished. Do not travel up spines uncast. I will live in you, until the next.


Come and play cards, and see who will win. Come and be the shadow in graves of misty acceptance. I am one to see things from where they came from. I am one to get lost, and then found again. I will not trip over myself, for any purpose.

## And for a Moment Everything Seemed Fine

There – look, there, in the window pane – a reflection – we don't see many like that. Not to be settled, though, in a movement. I have seen what others have not. And there, a likely pose, that wanders as it transgresses. Be calm – it will come.

Never springing forth – we mention names, names of the perplexed. And now we saunter, through and above. Do not linger now. Never linger. And in that we find ourselves in touch with more than ever. It is a touch of feigning.

A like-minded sort of thing that comes. I like it, so I will stay. And here, where the dance longs to be, there is motion, and a reclusive tread. I hear something profound – a silence in amongst silence. This will work, let us try.

Giving a loving glance, we see through what should have been. And then, like a rainbow that sleeps, waiting to be awaken, we walk that extra mile. My toes dip in the water, and I feel its coolness. Do wrap your fingers here – despite.

What we feel when it is not comfortable. What we feel when we transform this to that. When our lives improve via a simple transfiguration. Suffering, heightening, improvement. We will win this fight.

Clouds and all that will come to pass. I love what it is that keeps us going. I love the tentacles as they diminish. I love what it is that keeps us going. This much is seen by us. This much is captured. We will not give in.


Managing the ritual as best we can. Managing the running to all out accord. I sense a loneliness in these parks and gardens. Never one to diminish, I see things like never before. And here we find ourselves, without the mist to blind us.


A future event, we see, but cannot touch. There is now grease in the pipes – we will clean them. And here where the moisture is warm, we hear something deep within. It is here where we conquer, and know ourselves to be guided by fate.


Something that takes us places. Something that moves us. Something that harks back to our childhood. There is a movement here – from there to once again. Never feel yourself estranged from your past – it makes you, despite everything.


A whispering through the trees. Moonlight, and all that invigorates. We are in love with what we see, and see what we love. An embrace that does not disappoint. Come now, we must away from here. Let us go – and then? Aha, yes.

Instantaneous, like a feeling we never had. Living high, living deep. Caught in the fire, but not feeling the heat. I will be as I wish - and here, where strange things occur, I have recourse to the stars, and every little thing that counts.


What do we do when doing never helps? What do we say when saying only pleases? There is here something to share. There is here something in the air. There is now a walkway that has as its claim the morning and the twilight.


What counts as up, when down is all we seek? What is the vicissitude that will transform our lives? Sometimes it takes only one – only one, and let us raise ourselves. Let the height commence.


Having majesty, and being alive, there is now something we don't understand. I have not figured this part out yet. And here where the silence has taken us to the limit, a new found longing to replace the old. We will not fold.


A missing piece, one that harps in the lonesome steppes, like a renegade through and through. Be the barbs to our shawl, and what we will find will be bliss, and nothing more. I see the tempest – and I let it come.

And when we fly – we fly for good reason. And when we rest, we do also for good reason. Open the shutters, and let the light in. Open the gate, and the world will newly arrive. It is as if we had never breathed.


Treasure more than is thought, in all the books and all the history ever published. I will shake this before it becomes, by chance, the rumination of staid example, and what is next. Be the fire, it will not suit. Be the cooling balm. I will finish what is left.


In fairly good regard – what is this? Where do we go from here? There is a maelstrom that shoots fibres, down through the leggings, up into pieces. I have found what I was looking for. But what is that? There is time to tell.


A maestro of feelings. What comes when we are down? What eventuates when we have hit the bottom? Our consciousness heightens, and we simply ameliorate – we find what is needed. And transformation occurs. New found longing.


And then, like a web that holds no furry – then – we size up our belief, and send shards flying everywhere. That is what we can do – and that is what we will do - Launch into it – don't say a prayer, just vanish, and then come to.

## And for a Moment Everything Seemed Fine

Falling away – falling into dust and weavings. I sense your camaraderie. I sense your compunction. I sense what it is that keeps you going. And here, where the mystery never ends, we play at our feet, and know the dance to shed grace.

And now, like a window that looks onto neverness, there is a light that only shines in halves. And here, where we do not dread, here I sense your composure – there is time enough to sing a lullaby. But what comes next? We will envisage.

Nothing other than this. Nothing other than the fusing of winter delight. And then a rush of blood. I hear you now – hear you like never before. What is it that stops us? What is it that makes us cry? There will come a time when these things are set.

Giving what is more attuned. Catching the wave as it spills. We move ourselves like carpentry uplifted. I see your housing coursing. And now we are there. Do not bleed, we must only watch. And in this motion – anon.

There was a time, amongst all this, that we endeavoured to be in style, in the most deliverable way. When we had finished, sense, and the moving of cannonballs. I hear the gist of it in motions of light, motions of dark. We will continue.

If I have left, I have left with purpose. If I have dreamt, I have dreamt like sand. And when we have found our way from here to there – rations of the sky – just to see us through. I have never once thought otherwise – except in-between-wise.


Emotional pain – how is that dealt with by the suffering transformation? It is the same – the inner and the outer. Whenever we encounter pain which is inner, our consciousness heightens, and we transform, ready for life to improve.


And here, we have something we want to say. And that is this – We are born, we live, we die, under sway of forces unknown – but one thing is assured, we can overcome our suffering, and that is what we have at our disposal. We do not renege.


Floating by, on streams of liquid dreams. We have as a guide, all the sea can give. And then like a roundness, we have the sport that tailors all. Do not envisage the dance, it has only specs to harbour, and closeness to curtail.


Floating, on a wind that doesn't stop. Catching on turbulence – turbulence that does not stop. There is here something we cannot deliver. In the mystery of the tangent, here we seek ourselves. Much is thought of this – but here we go.


For everybody – for everything – listen, and you will hear a delight of the senses. You will hear it, and then it comes again, and then again, and then, without further recurrence, and in a matter-of-fact way, a hold – a holding on. There.


Figuring on things to come. Believing in what the sun stands for. And then like the trays that carry so much, we are there. Do not pretend. Do not waver. In these instructions is life – life unremitting. There comes a silence – it must.


When we hurt, we do so for our betterment. It just takes time. And there we have it. A semblance of the known and the unknown. Suffering goes up, and our lives improve. As a writer, that could be posthumously as well. Think about life.


And then like a rainbow, we step, and then, like a piece of land that denies all tropes. We are a mirror, a mirror to the sky, just like a still lake. There are no clouds in this sky either. We march, but to which beat? To which chorus?


Have the little we say, and bring it back on the fibres of the new and the old. Come and be part of the grand adventure of literature. There nothing like it. I will see myself in golden weave, and then like a fire on display, I will up the gathering.


Come my need – direct me where to go. Nothing can come from the beyond to harm us anymore. This is the staple and the curve. This is the stasis and the board. Do not trip, there are places to be and places to go. Shoot forth, and wonder with.


And now, like a shore-line approached, there comes a mission to be made. But what is it made from? What does it seek in adventure? I sense something I can only see. And then, like a barrage of life on life, there comes the message from afar.


Gorgeous, and ready to launch those thousand ships. Do not be the one to settle – the one to settle old scores. There is a window that looks, and in this look is the trace and the circumference. Chase, and be won. Chase – that is all.


Treasured deep. Forlorn but not forsaken. There is something new in each ruffled step. And then, like a cake that has never been eaten, we relish all that comes before. There is a likeness to the Pharos. We will sit and wait.


And then, with a punch of emotional pain (a punch only that pain can have), we see our lives getting better. Better already. And then, like the fibres of a

sea vessel, we see our measure, and take it.
Become heightened. Let your consciousness go.


And in-between, the this and the that, there
resounds a cry, a cry of sorts. And I know not what
else to say, but in this cry, is the carrying of ages.
There can be no other thing, that tempests are
hark to bring. Be without care, and you will be still.


To be the centre. Or rather, to be in the centre of
things, is to be at the quick and the marrow. I
know that what is left of us should not be shunned.
I know that what is left of us should only be used
for the purposes of worn out trying. We will
conquer.


What do we do that has not the simplest trace of
anything fresh. I sit, and am not perturbed. I
render, and am not at the coalface. I stand, but
only in the regularity of it all. And here, where the
signs sparkle, there envisages a trace of new
found longing.


Finding nothing to see. Finding nothing to be.
Finding all that is, and all that will be. I see, and
am not ruptured. I hear, but what of the cost? I
tumble, but do not bleed. And then, like ash on a
blanket, we call, and the response does not
diminish.

And now, without more than a whimper – we come again, like nuptials in further embrace. There is a chance at understanding, but we do not rely on finishing all the down strokes and the up strokes. Come and be, when being loves to be.


There is now a silence we cannot hear. There is now a worthy opponent. There is now the semblance of things done right. I will live for this, until trees fall down. I will live for the shade of it. Where no shadow is cast. Have no fear.


And now, where the dance is absolved, I will let my suffering fill me – fill me to the brim. And then, like a sustenance that prevails, there is time. In one motion, up, my suffering catapults in new directions – out and beyond, to what I need.


And then, like a shower of rain, we come, and see things for the harvest and the train. Do not sit still here, the drain casts its science across the yard. Do not belittle the stranger. He comes to say farewell. And like a tragedy, we are quickened.


I sense nothing else will come between us. There is a like-minded tangent in whatever we do. Come and be the solstice – we will rhyme. Come and be the lingering fast, as it shallows up to the window – we will see.

## And for a Moment Everything Seemed Fine

And like a tenacity that augurs truth, there comes
a willow in each hand. Willows that don't reside in
these parts. I hear your call, and know that the
sense of it has no boundaries. Can we fix the
moon so it does not shape? We will see.


Very much enamoured – we seek more. We only
seek what is left, and not of the horizon. Be that as
it may, the choice is simple. Come now we hark
back to the forest, and know the trading of blows
to be a farce and template. Yes.


What of this? What of the night? What of the sand
that keeps us grinning. We love to side-step the
wellness of it, and here rustle-up to the shore-line.
The co-mingling will never leave us. I hear my
heart, but not in the usual way. I will sit.


A last-minute dash – through the door, and out the
hall. I see you now, like never before. I see you
like a vast antechamber. Do not hesitate, there are
things to do, places to be. I have won at things,
but I will never hesitate.


What can suffering do? What can it give us, in the
meantime, and beyond? What we need, what we
want – Our approach to suffering transforms our
world. I will suffer, and sublimate, all the desired
things. Witness the flood, it will come.

A last marked hurricane. Twisting like flesh in amber settings. I see you, I see you now. It is as if the walls had come down, and the mischief of a fire creek had readied itself for the bleeding of day. Come now, let us commence.

There is an ambiance to it all. There is a letting of lives to the distance of the setting. I hear the last wish, and know it to be whole. There comes a maelstrom, but we are equipped. Do not herald the far away chime. It cannot hurt us.

I see much in between, much that harks a treat. But in the snow, we let ourselves go, and see that time is no enemy, and the vents of ashes are halved, and what is left cannot be one to the shelve of things.

What of the far-away? What of the recipe and the book? I hear your voice amongst things that only shine in willingness and the vine. There is a creed, in harrowing delight. I see it, amongst the embers of culture, and the witnessing of belief.

Hold on, the ride is slippery, and to the fold of it we come. Do not envision what is in this hold, for to do so is to bind ourselves to fate. I see you now, like embers on a lonely road. We love it here, where the starling never misses.

## And for a Moment Everything Seemed Fine

Without the need to try, we waffle in, and have our fill of life. And then, like birds on the rafters, we sit, and know temptation to be a thing of the past. I implore you, stand between this and that, and all that will transpire will hearten.

Even discomfort can heighten us. We hold on to things, and they rub. We change what we feel into reality. It is all in the way we see things. We transpose heart into daylight, into dreams. And then off we go – never to miss, nor be remiss.

Is this new? It is old. It is as old as people putting thoughts on paper. Do we dwell? Do we send the aforementioned steel to forests of clay? There is a mystery here that we seize upon. Do not rest ourselves away from it. Let it come naturally.

A fanciful way of it. I sense more than can transpire. Do you see the same thing I see? Do you cover yourself in ablutions? Never once have we seen this. Never once has the buried, and the tangent arrived so soon. We must wait.

Cordoning off what lies beyond. It is here where the difference begins to gather. Where the holistic benchmark leaves us together. I like what I see, see what I like. There is a feeling here we must not let go of – ever. Let us conquer.

And when we have come, we will come again, and then, even, once more again. There is little that can be done. Spendthrifts and delicate hearts. We know of no other way. Do we say what we need, and need what we say? Let us.

Again, I ask you – do you have the right tone of voice, the right inflection, so that we never look back? There are aces in front of us, and then behind. It is like we never were. Despite, there is a rousing crescendo. We will not listen to barbs. No.

How long, to be in or out of it? How long, to be in the throng? I have never met a lady by chance. I have never felt for certain what it is that keeps the metal pressed. I will have sight of traction delayed. There it is – yes.

I pucker up to the sentient embrace, and know that fire and ice never collide. I hear my voice, but what is the withstanding of it? My suffering is my suffering – it continually makes me anew. What will become of it? We shall see.

Clouds before dawn. Harkening for the rainbow to appear. I see much on my daily walk. I hear what cannot be heard. I sense like a father in renegade suns. Most of all I feel my pinions in dress of white. They take me places. They take me there.

And then, like a furthering of dread, we sense things that cannot be sensed. I touch what is never made for this. I long for the travesty of it to cease. But what is more, there are things that bind, and things that harbour no attention.

What is this motion that defies the night sky? What is this thing that runs by at speed? We have never believed for a moment that we could lie in wait, never for a moment. I see the gate, and I put heart through. What is left – who can tell.

I have a new mode, one that doesn't sleep. It curdles and sprays and listens like the wind. I know that this is not what we should be saying, but we must. There comes a reticence to believe. We never relinquish the right to dive. Dive deep.

Just for me. I guess these words are for joining. Cover up the sand, rituals burn for the love of it. There comes a time and a place for the reckoning of ages. Do not settle in, just yet. There is much to come, and much to become undone.

Testament to the knowledge. I hear the voice of it – it rings true. And now, like a fable that joins in for the retribution, there comes a rectifying motion. All hail the chief, and all come the wanters. I feel things like never before.

Hardship – there is time – time to mop the floor with it. We encounter it, and then we lift it higher – our lives get better – more full of whispered intrance. And now, like a burgeoning state, we see the life that we live, and we gauge it for more.


I am one never to see things in their roundabout state. I have as their void the gate of all absent wanderings. I see little. But what I do see rocks the life of it. I can do no more but look-on. And here, like a scape in dead of night – away, and through.


There is something I have yet to say – and this is it. If you are tethered through vines of green, vines of grey, unpick them, before harnesses come in fashion betrothed to order. And in this, we have victory. In this we have as the vastness reborn.


A vestige, one that has little to do. I warn you, do not waver, do not settle on the ship of castings. And now, I believe in one thing - and this is up and across. Come now, we do not foreshadow, nor alleviate, only to branch, and figure in rows.


I come, and believe in the journey. I see things as ripe, not as dull. I see things as rooved, and not what the train has to offer. There comes a token in marsh, and rising in straights of well-trodden ground. There is more to this – we will see.

## And for a Moment Everything Seemed Fine

I have as my reckoning all the style that each conundrum can bring. I look out the door for what comes next, and I see light, and treasures of faintest blue. There is here more that says hello. There is a jumping that has as its core the wishing well.


Much in line with things to do. Much in line with things to say. Much, and much. We seemingly leap forward, and know what is at stake. I hear what we believe, in rings of fibrous mass. And then, in time to things we wither up, and fasten ourselves in.


What do we call it when we hurt? What do we hear when things are astray. Our message is clear – suffer, and you will improve. That much is the way of it. I will, like no other, tend to wounds gone missing. Here, and here-abouts.


There is a gasping that has air as its residue. There is here, something more as well. What do we find when we look? What do we find when we saunter? There are lives and there are lives. We must, in turn, each one, not diminish.


Arriving, and then on solid ground. We have the most of what is next. We have the most that will always be. Come now, our vision is filled, we confront, and do not waste. I have the answer – it swims, and climbs on the debris of life.


I feel, but do not send. I have ardour, but not of the usual sort. And here, where the moisture of the fallow seeks in time to ingenious derivatives, there, there is much to follow. I will never linger more than is enough.


Come and be a part of the grandest play in the most secluded area. And now, despite the carrying of the day, there lives a giant of unknown proportions. I see myself in the greys and whites of it. And here, where we love to be, the choice.


Having what is said, and giving up all that can capture. There is a time, that harks, and is real. There is a mainstay, and the wrestling of tiny vertebrae. Be chosen, and what you will give will cast its lot in a chosen field. Do not delay.


Foraging for life – seeing where the noise will take us. And then, as in stillness, we gather ourselves for something sweet. I cannot tell where things are going. But that is okay, where we find ourselves is where we will end up.


A harrowing mass. When there is pain, there is release. When we move, we privilege, this over that. Our consciousness heightens, and that is for us. To be, where the few have gone. To lie still, where glaciers never render.


I need the height of consciousness now, to get me in motion. There is never any more to it than this. I need the suffering in my life. But I don't intentionally look for it – it just comes of its own accord. And when it does, I am there.


A lasting farewell. There comes a lingering by-play, that has as its ilk more than the pleasures of the past. We are honoured in what we do. We sound out what passes as regret, and know that the strangeness of the vicissitude ignites.


Come now, do you see? Do you see, as all of us? There is a repartee in the mile, and the semblance in the trade-off. Be warm, and the cold cannot frighten you. Be half, and the full will drive you to certainty.


What is this that we see? What is this that we feel? There is a limit to proceedings that have as its test the drive and the far-away. Do not rescind. Only when the trumpet blast has you. But that cannot be, and cannot be seen.


All the more. All the priceless and invigorating things in your life. There is a wonder, never about now. There is a catching of tales to tell. There is

never one to truly understand. But that is okay.
We will saunter, and then release.


There was once in front of us, the most harrowing
of responses. It was neither here nor there –
neither up nor down. Neither roundabouts, nor in
the circle. I will tell you what we are, and then we
must leave. Come closer.


And now, like a vacuum in summer sun, there
retains the eagle and the moss. I will come for the
chart, and have as the mistletoe all the vibrancy of
youth. I sit, and in this position I wait. There comes
a chance, and we must ready ourselves.


Pain and hardship – they give us much. They give
us the opportunity to improve our lives. What we
want, and what we need, and what can only be
described as the most precious adornment. Do not
linger here – the rough is at hand.


A semblance of the norm. I have in my ear, the
most tumultuous acceptance. And it is here that
we roam, and here that we consult the ardour of
our lives. Do not be the swallow in the swallow's
trance. Only sing once, and that should be
enough.


Come now, do you really feel that way? Of course,
a clasping in the mist. I sense your call, and issue

back your name. This is where sign posts rule.
This is where the falling denounces itself. I come,
and believe in strangeness. That much will be.


Often times we sit, and know the languor of the
mire to be a vast waste land. I have changed my
mind, a thousand times. And in those thousand
times are the shapes of a thousand wishes too
gently packed. I will not renege. Forwards only.


Gaining in strength – the thought we had has now
abandoned us. And then, like a ruin at dawn,
much to savour, and much to tender for. The hylic
and the bridge commence, never a one to shy
away, always a one to begin. Let us begin.


Which way to decide? Which way will we go?
There is something in each of us that burrows
deep. There is something that time cannot
pretend. I have witnessed much in my life, but this
is by far the most interesting thing. We will start
again.


And now, to sublimate. We wish and turn, and
have as our nearness the tide and its superlatives.
We turn dross into gold, suffering into something
else, something else that harbours such poise,
that it almost hurts. This is to sublimate.

Almond skin, and bristling mires. I hear your
fanciful applause in corridors of ancient night. I
see the arbour, and match it with the troop. Do
you see me when we are there? Is this part of the
play? There can only be what there is.


A fusion of light and sound. A boisterous
condolence that leaves a shear thrill. I come and
know my life to be at the vanguard of fate. I see
myself here, and then let go. Never once have I
seen the time it takes. But that is okay – we will
see.


Gaining in ambition, the lord of the place nears us
to completion. I sit, and am conscious of the
board. It tells us what time it is, and says only that
time is a bastion, and the wheels can only fall
through in unison to the rest of us.


Come and be prepared, there is a sense of the
jovial about it all. And now I sense a new
beginning, one that lies in wait, and snares, but
releases. There is something greater we must
speak of – and that is of the mist, and all she has.


Against it all, we search. Against it all we linger.
Against it all we pair back. This is the way it goes.
This is the way it tails. There can be only the well.
There can only be the way of it. I will tell of things
to come. And in this there is solace.

And for a Moment Everything Seemed Fine

Finishing the painting, it always takes a laugh. And then, in time to your favourites, a considerable meandering that leaves a touch of strength. That leaves a touch of wonder, through it all, and beyond. Do not flinch, more is coming.

Our combined suffering hears no sound, nor whispers in dead of day. All we must do is wait, and here it comes. Remember that it is powerful, and seeks no redress. We go higher, and in this state, we sow the seeds of our future. Yes, yes indeed.

Coming back – back on the flint of life. We hear what is next, and there is a shudder before we can stop ourselves. We must wander here, wander in staunch acceptance. Acceptance of what is, and what will be.

I am singing to the which-way hooray. And it is here where the night is languid and not at all solid. We hear ourselves in majesty, and in hope. Do not catch the rhythm, there is no time. I wonder what is left – this or that?

I see what it is that holds us back. It is something quite special, and in need of something else. We can change it to what keeps us going, and in that we will never remonstrate. Come for the life of it, and come for the ceiling. You will not be sorry.

A commotion, and then light. We see ourselves in the average, and then beyond. Do not find us lacking. Do not find us strewn. And here, where the master of the place gives a grievance – here we will frolic on sand dunes made of the sea.

Sorting out our lives, we catch a hold of the temerity and lift it high. There is now a time to be in spades of red, spades of colour. And then like a random appeal, we consider the luck of the brave, and the staunch, but unremarkable, setting of things.

Justifying the causes. Feeling in harmony with the measure. I know of no other way. And then, like a stable, with doors ajar, we let ourselves wander, and then come back once again. This is no picturesque development. It just is.

We must just let our suffering enfold us. And in that embrace, between this and that, these are the seeds of a larger turning. A turning that we never thought possible. Up, and away. Through and beyond. To a new life, one that sings as it sheds.

And now, in-between the chisel and the mace, we sculpt a new figure, one to last a thousand years. There comes a panacea, to right all wrongs, and give what is hardest most attention. We are through, and out, and we belong.


But what of the mix, of the dirt, and snow, and accumulated weatherings? I will build myself a chamber, so that I might see the daylight anew. Is this what we hope for? Is this what we say? Holding on, we canter, and know the languished tide to be.


And when we emerge, we do so with a strength that casts its shadow further than before. With an ease that parries nothing else better, we long for the strangeness of it to return. And, when we least expect, a towering, one that does not belittle.


Fascinated by it, we trudge on, and go deeper than ever. It is as if we had not seen the door of it. And then, like a fire that cannot cast. Like a runaway that does not scold. And like all things – embraced by the steepness of it. This comes to the fore.


Disappearing, but with trace. There is a round moon, that doesn't ensnare. There is a catechism, to be held in brief, and then like a rain shower, to diminish with time. Come now, open the door – it stands the test, and then, more.

Much to say – much to enjoy. And like a spark that doesn't render, here the faculty of the heart moistens. Is this what we have come to expect? Is this the lay of it? Is this what we have come for? I hope, in time, we will see things around.


Incredulity, and the mischief of the stars. I know how much of this is left. I know how straight the glacier is. And then, like a time that comes in droves, we listen to the trees in the forest, and know them to be calm. That will suffice.


What comes at us, is not what we expect – suffering comes in just this way. We must adapt, and let our natural faculties rise, and tender a new dimension to revel in. We can convert – this to that, and create a life in the middle. Yes – time on.


Foraging, and placating. Laying waste, and then not wasting. A belief in every small thing. A couch in the city. A couch, roundabouts. We love what it is that we see, and we see what it is that we love. Come now, there is no tom-foolery here.


What the dance never lets go of. What we are not ashamed to believe. What trickles down the rose-cheeks, and gives the semblance of laughter. What we can only see in the way, on our journey there. There is like something never before seen.

A rapid that seems more difficult than it is. Consternation in the crowd. A full and dextrous approach. This is the way we call ourselves. This is the way we tend to our lot. And then, intransigence, and all that will come to be.


What more do we think about these things? What more do we have to say? I will not let the commotion cease, only in time to a chosen view will we ever stop. And then, even then, we can never relinquish. It is continued in the vastness of it all.


Forbidden, but entrenched – allowable, but never decided. I come for the forebears, but diminish in reluctance. There can only be what we miss, and here where the sound of cobblestones reaches, there is a chance at height, and all it will bring.


What do we say when we find water? Is it the same as what we say when we find reverie? This is true in many ways. This true in one way, at least. This is a truth to be betoken. And now, linger I can't. For in this, life resides.


Suffering – we encounter it, all we do is knead it like dough, and make something of it. And then in the sense that arises, we lay the planks for a new type of life. One rounded with the spoils of adventure clad. This much will take us.

What do we see in the vale? What do feel in its embrace? What is the camp set for? Do we really know what we are going for? This is a tendency, one that grows as it softens. I heed no call, and retrench no barb. To this we say a mighty, 'triumph'.

Forging ahead, we now know our destination. It is here amongst it, and around the troupe. Dovetail, and see what comes. Dovetail, and litter the roadway with dreams. This is what it is all about. This is what most tingles on the spine. Yes, and again.

A hotchpotch of feelings – but only one is given in motion, and in sense. It is here we send the royal of society into due course. Come now, do not boast. The things we hub, and never what we need at any-rate, are the things that never list.

Coming for a caption, we adore what it is that we see. And then, like never knowing which way to go, we turn ourselves around, and have what is left arch the Mary-fantastic. Come now, time will tell, and times often do. Yes, indeed.

Caught in-between this and that, between whole and half. There remonstrates a demon of far-off denouncing. There is here a nuance, that blisters in new time, new feeling, and new resolve. There will be a tether loosened. One to choose by.


I catch what it is that holds me back. I see what can never be seen. I hear, what only has a wall to cry against. I love what cannot be told otherwise. Do not tend to the bricks and mortar, there is something here that bites. We will trudge.


Gaining in solace, we hear our sides diminish, and know the rendering of steel to be a boon and a blessing. Do not stop now – we must not only continue, but we must thrive in this world. Come and be part of this amazing adventure.


Fasting to play right, fasting to see things through. I have a mind to sit with dis-ease and know friendship to be the tidier of all things. There is hope, and a small degree of discomfort. I will not let this linger. It has to have an end.


Come and wish for the easier of two options. Come and be what the dance is supposed to be – the loom is supposed to be. And then, like rain of a tin roof, there is a quarter of a mystery remaining. We hold on – hold on for dear life.


Having the courage – being quite summoned about it. And then like an aegis too small, we spring forth, and desire nothing more. I sense something of value here, I sense something of heart. And then, like now, we suffer - and raise it up.

Caution, caution to the sail – it unfurls quickly, with speed. And then, like a touchstone, we are away, and in mode. I sense something else here. I sense the tide and its strength. I sense the ravages of the night, and all who pass in slumber.

Sentimental, and indicative. We search, and then find. We cable, but for which assortment. There are rungs we do not allow. But here the fabric is torn, and the test of wills comes in staunch regard. There will be time, I know it.

Up, goes our suffering – up and through, and then beyond. Into things we can close on. Into things we have made – into things we choose upon. And in that, there is a merriment, one that does not sting. We have found a way. But what now?

Everything is still. Everything wanders. Everything has a place. Just this, I hear you say. Just this. And now, like a candelabra that has no mission – like a vision in dead of night, we come, and are not circumspect. We listen, but to where?

Everything is on fire. We hold on, but where does the light come from? Where are we sold? Can there be a proper time, a proper enthusiasm, and all that is not remiss? I see you now – like a gorge par excellence. It will be.

I see your plan, and I raise you a raft of velocities, of velocities gone that way. And here, where the sound of the sea lulls us, we walk forward that little bit quicker. But what are we for, this trench and I, we capture, and then trundle. Yes.

An automated thing, one that does not rush, nor have time to navigate. This a partition of the soul. This is where we come to, when we are lost. And then, like a magic, we disappear – but then return, with added strength.

Envisioned, and draped, we are enthralled by what goes on. There is a tenderness that harks to no man's heart. And this is where we linger – right to the very end. We cannot grasp the tenacles of this. We will simply wander.

Withdrawing, and not alone. We seek what it is we need. We harbour what the night will give us. And then, as is mentioned in the pamphlet, there will come a time for change. A minuscule event, and something to take us there.

What can lift us higher? What can invigorate us such that we never come down? Hardship, and the embrace of time. There is a wind here, going from north to south. But also from ground to sky. This is our future. We must embrace it.


Ballooning, and transcending. Never a moments rest. We come, and are gone. We live, and do not regret. It is here we find ourselves nestled, and in love. In love with the journey. We do not speak in tongues. We only speak to the regions.


There is a place for this in the sun. There is a place for this in the sand, the sand of centuries past. What have they managed, what have they caught between steel fibres? This is something we cannot trample. Something we cannot fear.


Every moment of this is fine. Every moment of this can embark. What we sense, we have not lost. What we dream, we have only encountered again. There will be a sound from within. And with that, we lose ourselves in fun and adventure.


Having to stretch to move around. Having to guard against the levity of all situations. There is something in this we never believed in before. But that is okay, the remedy is here. We uphold ourselves to the festive light, and feel the cheer of dandelions.

## And for a Moment Everything Seemed Fine

A sort of rectilinear motion, one that does not surprise. We catch what it is that is left of our lives, and sprinkle it down through the ages. And then, like a forerunner to fate, we hold on, and see the best of us as it continues in vast array.

Finding out what things are all about. Loving the life, but not giving in. Having the speed and wherewithal. Never minding what. I come, but do not beseech. I linger, but not on common ground. There is a fence around proceedings.

What is never left behind, is a good piece of suffering. We eat it up like a fine breakfast. It means our future is bright, and our consciousness gives height. That much is offered in solace and in spring. That much.

Languid, and disarmed. We halt for major shifts in tendencies at a stroke – a stroke of the pen. Do not say 'strangeness', to a stranger in a strange land. There is an effort here, not to undo. Not to undo the traipsing of wrestling with the eagle.

Come now, there is no opportunity like this – anywhere. There is no place like here, no time like when. And then, in harvest, and in shine, we know which way to go. In harvest and in shine. This much we know.

Almost rattling, almost caring too much. There is a vigour here, a vigour towards the template. Do not curtail, the seeming and the trawl. I know of much that will suffice. Much in the offing, much in the land of it.


Contrition, and the reminiscing. Off-beat, and insecure. We hope now, not for the cold of winter, but for the rough of summer edge. There is more than is possible. There is more than the night. We will uphold the day (for what it is worth).


I look beyond, and I see what can only be seen in fairy tales. It is here, where the mouse and the elephant display, a mutual cry is heard, and tenacity and insistence begin to flourish. I will not harbour a grin. Not for anyone.


Living in an estuary of thought. Breathing like we were never encumbered. I fall – but then I rise. I believe in things, but then am collided. What is more, I sense the way of it, and am placated. There is time to be, and time to rush. We will find.


A vicissitude comes, and we let it. Here is the way forward. We open, and let the draft in. Our consciousness goes higher, and then we bring things into our lives from a far. We manifest what we need. And that is not anything dispensed.

## And for a Moment Everything Seemed Fine

Having more than the tempest. Dreaming in a far-off state. Dreading nothing of what we have. There brings something of the wilderness. Something of the suture. Something of the brochure. And then, that the willing are the glad – we fly.

Arranging things so that they don't get in the way. Arranging things so that the air remains taught. Come now, don't fashion a rung of it. There is a place for this in the master stroke. Something we see, but must not tantalize. What for?

Glee in the face of it. Smart and for the neutral and the brave. What we encounter cannot be one and the same thing. This is what we fight for. This is what we read for. This is what it is for. And then, like a kaleidoscope, fusion - fusion without cladding.

A flagship circumference – lights that shine. A testament to the range – we hope we will never find it. To believe once again. To have the throwing of stones. To not have the tenderness we seek. Not to displace the horizontal with the vertical

And then, fanning aside the mysteries of the land, we are one to sell ourselves again – like a surgeon in the way of it. We conquer, but for what purpose? We drool, but for what exposure? There comes a rapid-fire movement. We will brace ourselves.


Nothing left to give. Nothing left to say. Hardened by the journey, we have more in the way of it. Come now, do not faulter. Come now, do not stray. There is fire in this room. There is fire in this alley. We laugh, but what holds us? We will see.


We come. We are pronounced sensible upon arrival. There is never more than this. There is never less than more. Our suffering propels us forward. Up and across, Up and across. New ways of living present themselves. We have won.


A sky that does only fall. A listening that guides the wayfarers. Holding on, we grasp at straws, and know the life of it to be true. Carrying on. Being delectable and entrenched. Solitary, and yet not victimised. A reef of snow.


Having to hold on to things, but not believing the distance succumbed. I hold each pattern in my hand like a trolley exposed to the rush. And then, like a bird on its first flight, we see the magic of movement soaring through. Yes, indeed.


Hurrying to avoid the rain. We have no umbrella. Hurrying to avoid life – no, never. And with the aegis on things to come, there is a message to be heard. Write now, consider later. Something of the jam inside the jar. Carry up.


Gaining in strength, we forward ourselves towards the arrow, something that speeds passed us anyway. There is now a time and a place to hide away. We will take it, and then emerge once again. Fishing for pearls. We have flight, but more, we have fight.


Having the drawing of past endeavours, having the sun like a radiance of trees. I evoke, and then tremble. I see, and then relax. I hurt, but only in the wind. I trample through, only to gain attention. Do not see the way as it stands – it is here.


Gaining in direction, we gather pace, and a new found calm. What is here? What do we seek? There can never be anything more like this. I am wanting to dig the dirt around me, so that I can escape the tethers that bind. Be willing, and find.


I ask myself to take on more, and rejoice at the being. I know of nothing more delightful than the can that holds us – than the wire that lets us go. In the meantime, there is play, and a certain frolic, to be had – to be had by more than we.


The sea is rough. But what commissions the board? What commissions the day? There is nothing like this in all the world. There is nothing like this here and now either. I will petition the part of me that wavers – and fix it to the dawn.


I love what it is we do. I love this part, so very much. But then, like a harbour in waiting, we feel the rush of it, and know like a wind in mourning, that the signs are good. I can see no negative on the plain. No recourse to delivery.


Come and be quiet. There is a makeshift attendee, a thing that holds on que, and knows the wind to be a solace. We love, but who also loves for us? I know that the distance round-a-bouts is not something we can salivate at. Here we are then.


A caution, a caution to the tempest. There can only be that which we launch. And here, there can only be what the dime says is here for striking, and not for naming. I have once said to the canvas, you cannot touch me.


There was once a start in a cave of unknown strength. And here, where the whistling and the set of branches do not speak, there comes a mountain of salt to dish and to remember. And like so much more, there comes a favourable wind. We will scatter.

Dreaming, but from afar. Yawning, but to which vantage? I hope nothing in-between loves this is as much as I do. The falconry estate feels just right. The method we have entangles. But what of it? We will proceed. And then?


Forming an opinion – giving what is not a question. Being able to stand – for the quarter at least. I have in me something that doesn't cater. But here, where the sand is recondite, we blister a way forward – like time itself. We will come.


Come this way, we see all that arches. And like a sky that harbours no ill-will, we carry ourselves forwards, in time to an applause that knows when to erupt. I have a feeling of camaraderie with shivers down the spine. Wait, it is in tune.


A vicissitude awaits. And in that, a movement for and against. And what we find brings us to our knees. We suddenly have what we need. Up and beyond. Never a thing left behind. We can't wait. We can only cast a shadow at the dawn.


Formidable, whilst burning bright. Encased, encased in snow. There ruptures a unison that has not the pleasure to feel. There ruptures an event that races to the line. Be like we may, there is a chance to harvest at the finish.

A sycamore, one that treats itself well. One that
harbours something clean to the touch, and sans
emotive structure. I listen, and I know what is next.
I know the fire has been lit, and it now burns in
untold ways. We will let it.


Constant, and approving. Deleterious to the touch.
We send our selves through each gate, without so
much as a care. Do not pretend, how life and love
can intertwine, so much for the harrowing of it. We
will bend, until the chime of it ceases.


Getting through, and in ample time. Getting the
most delectable motion. Forwarding things
around, and then going ahead. There rings a
sense tantamount to being low. But this is not that.
I have never believed in things like this.


Vicissitudes. What do they teach us? What is their
store? They come, and are laden. Laden with
what we want and need. Do not seek them out,
they will come. And when they do, rejoice – treat
yourself, and then see them run.


I sense something here, something more of the
tenderness of things. Do not frolic on wasted land,
it pangs to remember, that what is left is not for
the carriers of signals to portray. This is written in
sheaves, and a more triumphant ring.

## And for a Moment Everything Seemed Fine

What does the artist tell us? There is pain, sometimes emotional. We seek redress, and have it at our touch. Their work expands, on the senses, and renews its core to the centre of things. A piece of larder hangs merrily. We will enjoy.

Never like this before. But that is fine. That is the way things go sometimes. And then, like a passion in sunlight, we find new breath, new seeds, and new elongations of the marrow. What is this? Solace, and the chirping of lullabies.

Fixing on que. Flexing with might. We are the ones ready to soar. Never has the mind been so susceptible to so much. But when we find ourselves, that becomes the way of it – in tune, and without regret. See us now – we will ablaut.

Gaining the strength to carry on. Having what is needed most. Being archived, and then believed. What we at first remember of things. What it is time to do. What we force ourselves to consider, and then never renege.

Having the need to escape the bind. We are here, and we will listen. Caught in time to our chosen wandering. Be that as it may, we temp our shores along blissful avenues. Come and be the way of it. It will sing.

What lore is this? What is the chamber of delight?
We agonize over our suffering, but it lets us be
free, and to have the courage to transcend the
everyday. We must not seek out suffering though
– let it naturally come. It is yours.


And then, like a time that never was. Like a sand
that beats in the way of it. There augments a
temporary assailing, one which we are capable of
dealing with. I will not look back. I will not stop for
the rain nor the travesty.


This is where we begin. This is where the tempest
now has no bite. No room to move, nor no sound
to vanish. I hear the best of it through the awnings.
And here much room to see in slides of day,
debacles of another moment.


I see what is new. I see what is old. I come for the
way it shines, and the way it diminishes. Do not
believe in one thing after the other, there remains
a tutelage to the dawn. Have faith, there is
warmth. There is a cavalcade to sort through.


And now, what do we say? What do we say to the
moon, a saying that doesn't crumble. Let's
inaugurate it. Let us see what can only be felt. Let
us drown out the noise, and know it to be
something of the past.

## And for a Moment Everything Seemed Fine

Let us now transition to the clime that has as its border the nothing of the lyre. I sense the broom and the swept, as they frolic in new found reverie. Do not let go of the ground beneath your feet. It holds you there, and can never let you be.

There was once a knowing that had as its tenor all the shards of glass ever stood upon. But here, where the sound of being stands in reluctant surmise, there is accustomed, a fire bright array. We stand for nothing less.

What is it that keeps us moving? What is it that keeps us alive? It is all of this, and all of this alone. Without it, we distance, and slowly and utterly demise. Come now, do not feel the wanting for the wanting embrace. Feel it now, it hums.

And now, we listen – listen with hearts open. And it is these times that we shed, and try not to let the wind in. There is a temper that has no ilk of what it can actually be. And then, like a force of nature, we come.

All the furrowed brows, seek in themselves that desire of release. And when we can no longer speak, we utter a cry, that betokens all the harvests of all the lands. There is a battle cry that seeks no injury. It is here like never before.

And in the gloom, a spark is made. For a brevity, it lights the dark, and has as it temper an arrangement of sorts. There can never be anything like this – anything like this in all the world. We must praise the water – it is littered with gold.


I have in the shape of my consolidation a newly formed and nape arrangement, that harks in solid tones to what the dying of transmission will want to levity. I sing, but what for? I treasure, but which delight? There is an aloneness we seek.


Flying forward, we temper ourselves in new gained surmise. And when we are done, we arc the arches straight. There can never be a slow baton – one that brings us in from the world. I itch my back, as in a solemn rite to be.


Willows in the sun. Racing forwards to catch the last of it. We hide, and then re-appear. We guide, and are guided. I like what it is I see. All is in readiness. The ark contains all. There can only be what we seek. There can only be.


I drive the course, and have as an infatuation more than is necessary. Come and be placated, there is nothing more like it. Dreaming of the stand, we come in the dimensions of stillness. And what we have seen will surprise.

## And for a Moment Everything Seemed Fine

In the afternoon, we haze about with amazement. During the journey, there were times we feathered the rail with aplomb, and knew no other way to station the need nor the rainbow. This sounds like intuition, but is rather exalted. We will stand.

Knowing of no other way, we sit, and let our release be in time to so much. I have never envisioned the roughness of all that passes for the stand and the reign. I love this part, where things come together, and know that they will never part.

There is a set place for all that carries weight with it. I am at a loss to find the coriander with the soup. Do not appraise what cannot be appraised. Do not rescind what is stationary. We see the view, and know that things are righted.

An aggregation, of sorts. A feeling like the strands of it were put there to be played with. I sing, but I cannot curse. I love, but only so that I can stand. And then like a movement in the sky, we take notice, and send the aftereffects ploughing.

Nuances, and the right form of diagonal living. We stand ourselves in the way of it, and then remember which way to go. There is time enough. There is something else. We can't seem to abide the change. But that remains all and reclusive.

Withstanding. Holding what releases. I find you marking time. I find you seeing twice. There is a magnificence in the air. There is a bark in the breeze. It reckons forth, and in that juncture, finds itself anew. What is this, I hear you ask. Something quilted.

At this point, all we need do is stipulate, and posture new recall. We suffer, yes. But in that is something deeper. We call to the light of day – what can we do? What can we say? We can do all, we can say all. We sublimate, and turn things on their ear.

Having the speed of foot to mark the time it takes to rattle the bones of infinite jest. But what is so surly about this? There is a tension in ancient places. Not when the dance is cast in bronze. It is like the fabric of things resides in more.

We clash our way forward, and in that have as the stasis of things to be awakened. I love what it means to sense a valve in measure of the lead. And now, like cheese on bread, we no longer fumble, nor entrance our compartment.

Have it there, have it in the recipe of times on times. You must not set your hand at the fusion of lattice-all embarkments. This is how this cascades. This is how things never run. Never have the chances been so bright.


I am fortunate, I can see the way as it stands. And then like a far-fetched encounter, we travel. We travel, and feel no lack. What has become of us? We stride forth now, with a strength that harks in angel's breath. This will find us.


Closer, and then together. We measure all that is in turbulence. We seek all that is in endeavour. This is like the last stop on an ethereal train. And here we see ourselves in a long-lost pose. What should we be? What should we play? We must.


A major insistence, one that also alleviates. I do not deviate from the path of sparse remembering. But here, where we have cried so much, there remains a truth to be had. Where we file away the deepest – there can only be this.


What is suffering anyway? Why do we need it? We need it to build new lives for ourselves – new vistas – and new calming balms. There was once a dragon fly that knew how to fly. And like a rose in bloom, we kept sailing.


Saddle up your horse, the journey is just commencing. And when we finally come to the end, new walks will straddle the divide. What is

here, is not there. What is there is not here. Come
and be the standard bearer.


Having room enough to keep the motion going.
Having what will never depart. Always dragging in,
never out. And in the gloom, a space. And in the
gloom a sprint of light. One that forwards can keep
in the palm of its hand. Yes.


A mask that outshines. A masquerade that sees
all faces. I sense a new found absolute, one that
partitions the void, and goes on climbing down the
well. There is now a temporal adjustment to be
had. Let us have it.


Coining a new phrase – let it rhyme – let it have
assonance – let it have alliteration – but also, let it
refer to suffering, or some aspect of it. What clears
the way. What arrows in naught. I will tell you
again – do not faulter. This much will get us there.


There is now a way of shores. There is now a way
of envelopes. I see you there, like a tree in winter
– a tree painted by Tom Roberts, or Arthur
Streeton. There is something more we must
consider – and what is that? We will see.


Sometimes, in the wake of it, there is a cauldron –
one that relishes no fear. We laugh, and have as
our study more than the twinkle that forbids. What

is this now? Harlequin dreaming. And a source of
the tributary. We will dissolve.


What does it mean to suffer? What does the valley
say? There are many ways to find it, but should
we last and say it is all diminished? This is the
way, let us not tarry. I type, but where are the
letters? We will believe in more than has dotage.


But what is it that we can do? What is it that
seems to scent? We will never lay down. We will
never. And in that motion, a fabric that desires no
tinder. A compassion that sits in grounds of joy,
grounds of detail. And like things now, we
acquiesce.


What are the signs of it worth? Do we praise the
embers, or sit for the recalcitrant? We never vary
our invectives. We come for the stationary, and
listen in close. I am signed out – signed off. I will
only be what can be. Watch and stare.


What is dissolute, is not in the antechamber. What
is dissolute, is only pinched twice. I am the thing
that is recondite. Much, and so, tempting. What is
in the rain of it? – We purchase, and are tamed.
We don't see the train.


Are we gathering of pace? Are we the temptress
and the dial. Do we embark upon a journey of no

consequence? Never. Do we exclaim our voice to
line of it? There envisages more than commotion.
I love what we see. What we see is great.


Bursting, bursting through. There are no shambles
– at least at this point. We call to be the tether,
and not the sham. Victory is in the heart of it.
Come now, hold on. We are the ground beneath
your feet. This will always reckon.


And when the need we have convinces us that the
further we go, the better – here we will not stand
alone. Forging for the tenacious, we arc the solo
climbs, until twisted tree branches renews our
vows, and sends us once more to the brink.


But what of the vicissitude? It can help. It can
show its way down backs of utmost ardour. We
simply must let is do its work, and we are there.
Do not dream otherwise. Do not let the door to
frozen waste open.


And when we wind in, there is a time for tempest's
past. I see much in this way. I see much, and then
little. What can the dogged and street urchin say?
What we say has the mind set of the worker bee,
and all that clasps in dead of night.


Be the stable door through the weaving of things.
Be what can only be in fairy tales. There is a test

to delimit what is possible. There is a ransom to
be paid – but it does not resemble the far and the
wide. Think in wonderment.


Giving necessity what it is worth. Finding the
median point, and following. Causing a flutter, not
like the rest. I will be tempted by nothing less. And
when we are at the brink, and there is nothing left
to do – here, oh here, is where we find ourselves.


A sound in the alley way. A noise in the park.
What is gracious enough can only harm us from a
distance. Do not stray, stray over bridges of
tumult, bridges of abandon. We will hear what is
loud and clear. This is told of us.


Gesticulating, and wandering, what is it we seek?
What is it that the warrior bride holds? I sense
something in the window. It is here we get our
inspiration, and our preparation. In this we cry
tears of the sky, tears of day. Never whisper.


I have found a way through. Not through the
night, but through into the air. Visitations are a
wholesome bet. And then, like a credence that
doesn't differ, we emerge from our slumber, and
find, just like before, we find ourselves aloft.


When we suffer – something twigs. Our
consciousness goes up, and after a time, our lives

fill. They will fill with what we need and want. The more intense the suffering, the greater the effect. Sometimes we must wait. Sometimes like a poet.


Holding the jar aloft. Holding what the equation means. Being enraptured, but not sitting still. There is a turn of pace here – we see it. And with heart and soul we participate in the larger drama. There can be only what we think.


Never be one to attribute the tributary with what defies. There can only be some more that we do, that keeps the daylight happy. Do not distil the plains, and have the launch of the steady and the brave. Come – but do not be convoluted.


Fishing for the heard. Being the sign of it. Being instilled. A fabric that remains un-named. What is here, can never really be here. What is lost, can never be relinquished. I love what this is. I love to stand and wait.


Grass in the garden. Grass on the lane. We set foot on forever, and have the past of it rear, and then, you are there. Much is said, and much is unsaid. We have the like of it smiling, batting, and all out being a circumference to so much.


A future that doesn't compare. A round of recourses. And then the middle of it. And then something that pledges, pledges as it winds. I see you now, amongst all that which facilitates. It is here I know you best. It is here I know you.


What is this for? I hear the question, but what is the answer? In the fold of exquisite dilapidation, there gives a promising laugh. And it is here where the dimensions of the square lie perpendicular to the sun. We will see the dregs of it.


What is beneficence to the window? We hold our tongues, and have the food we eat come in solemn acceptance. I ring for the hourly ritual, and know that screens will never give way. I am looking at the oval now. What do I see?


My suffering knows only that it is there. The rest is up to me. I must grasp it, and send it once again home. But my reward is to sit in the middle of a time full of genius, and see it flourish like the wind. Be the source, and you will be strong.


There rises a chain. It does nothing, but rise. We see it and have as the touchstone a life to lead. We delineate the time of past encounters, and know that yours is in the way of it. Do not punish yourself – harbouring doubt is not you.

Affixing the line to the causeway, we do not cross. And then without the slightest conundrum, a new beset to cast off the old. It is as if the sand has been taken, and let go in a cruel wind. I love this part in any adventure – here we go.


Causing more than is dressed to see through, we consider our options, and then pounce, right on top. It is here where the volume of disguises embarks on every possible way. Do not have as your companion whispers to stars on stars.


A sense of relief. But for what, for what do we disseminate? Clouds hang, but do we act for them? – In some cases yes, but often no. I am the past, the present and the future. But what climes inside us, is every bit as tremendous as the sky itself.


Corresponding with the arrows of it. Being moved, but only forwards. Coming through, but then coming down. Afterwards we tarry. Afterwards we sing. But here where the fantasy of life beckons, here, there is more to say, and more to do.


Overarching, but still feeling it. There is a pleasure in this, oh lofty one. But do not feel the pulse of things left undone. I treasure the time it takes. And here, where the mystery of it all is clearly written, we have a chance to really acclimatise.

And for a Moment Everything Seemed Fine

Suffering – it cannot win. We have you now, so nothing can invigorate you further. There is something this move takes, and it is a solemn cry in the chamber of the heart. In this, a stroke of masterful intensity. This is us.

Finding the road, and seeing it meander. But that is what we have, isn't it. A sense that the crisp highlights of the sanctioning breeze are never one's to move. I will take no lounge with me. I will take what I have, and seize upon the window for help.

Have no fear – The roundabout is here. Have no fear - what wishes itself in time to the climb of it will always be there. A tackle to the place of it. A tackle to all that comes. We have heard what is in the trees – and it is you.

Forever, and then, what is more – a trace. A trace that follows the sky. We are nearing what is left. We are nearing what surmises. I will have dinner ready for you. And then, a long-lost opining that beckons to the undulations of an age – Yes.

A fog, that only moves, very, very slowly. Something to cast off, and then return to. Something that has as the embers of proclivity just sitting there. I hear your voice, but wonder as to mine. This is what makes it, and what makes it chuckle.


Mounting, and scything. Coming full circle. I will not wait, for anything, nor the dam. I sense a way to encapsulate – more than is enough. I will caravan with people I know, but only in the summertime. For then it is worthy.


Only coming into now. Only drying up the tears now. Only forging the way through. I have felt like a cinnamon tale, I have known all that is to be known – but still I come back to the tempest. There is a lark beyond measure. We will find it.


Suffering, I can hardly speak. But we must have it, and when we do, there is a change of heart, and a place to relate to. I know of no other way, but here and beyond. Come now, we must not pretend. This is where we are at, and where we will stay.


A little bit of heart, and more of the same. I have what we encompass, and know, that in the meantime, much is found on the path, and much besides. I sense what it is you need, and that is more than a tailor can brook.


Slow at first – and then gaining in speed. There is a time for the menagerie to find its peace – peace of mind, peace of life. I have heard, like an ember in dreaming, that what we give, gives itself a radiance of hope – radiance of joy.


There is a fundamental opinion that riles as it is kind. There is a belief, once there, is always there. And then, like a fog on a mountainside, it comes. Like a crouching shadow, we move, and are never relinquished.


Forming what is not an option, we linger, and then embark. I see the chance of it written in the wind. But how do we do that – write on the wind? With imaginations as strong as steel. With minds as condensed as ever. This will not smart.


Straight to the point. We love, and are moved. We soar, but with iron wings. We hear, but what is the motion? There are things we simply do not understand – but there are things we do (more importantly). Whisper, and trade blows.


There, in the distance, there, there is light. But how do we get to it – we suffer, and raise our suffering up. What we seek is not an adjustment – but the fundamentals. What we each know can fill a mountain pass. This will come in handy.


Belonging, but not settled. Placating, but not at a time. Being dishevelled, but still enamoured with the world. I feel a breeze. It comes in small mists, and does not curtail itself to the centuries old display. I will linger no more.


A gust – we feel it, and are sent to the rim of it. I see you here, watching and waiting. I see you here, amongst the flutters. There is now a chance to see what will come. See what is in the moorings, and what is of the tribe. Aplomb.


A weaving that does not hesitate – hesitate for any man nor woman. I feel the invective to move, and then I languish in simple strides, simple measures. How are we directed? Through passion, and the lease on the veritable.


Hold on, there is still time. Hold on, the trees are here to still. We feel it, and only it, through the shafts of blindness, and the overbearing arch. Constantly we arc, and then, as a ranger to be, we straddle the divide, and sing a laugh to see.


Having the stoic inside us to never let fall. A beautiful gesture, one encased in gold. There comes something special, something that is never uprooted, nor never as spontaneous as we think. A well in the vastness. We will go there.


Magnification, alluding to the time that is left. I hurry in, as we all do, and have as the asking price, nothing that falls short. Be pleasant, and we will all beckon. Be the tome, and watch the lights expand in front of our very eyes.

Consistent, and through much endeavour, we depart in gales of wonder and directed ease. Do not find the renegades trodden. There is left here something that cannot be wasted. There is left the pleasure of it all. Come and be served – it will suit.

What do we find when we suffer? Sometimes it seems insurmountable. But when we get through it, here is the rub. When we get through it, things get better. Thanks to our heightening of consciousness, we simply manifest what we need from life.

A long way to go. What we can only see is the way before us. I sense ablutions in the future. But what are they anyway, apart from the dream and the sleep. I hinder nothing, and I am free. I listen, but that is what guides me. Never mind.

Come now, do not retort, there are visions on the stairwell. There are places we love, and things we need to do. I think as much as I can. I will write until I am dead. But then, the hope of a nation rings true. This much we have learnt. This much.

Alive, and living. There is a constant approbation in the weave of it. There is something we have

never been told before. There is now a light
behind the blind – all we must do is lift it up, and
we can see. Do not hold back either.


A slight embrace – something that before now has
never occurred to us. I love, and cascade, and
have as the score a touching moment, one that
scales the heights, and sinks in. I know of nothing
else like this. I will give it my best.


A mainsail that creeps in harbours blue. A sense
of right that just seems to grow. What we hold, in
our hands, is something that cannot be curtailed. It
is of much needed gain, and much remembered
salt. Do not collide here – we are with.


Our suffering does not envision another fate. It
only comes for us. But when it does, we will be
ready – what do you want to do with your
suffering? There are chasms that can easily be
gotten out of. And here, fate, and the wheel of it.


Growing in stature, we have as our breeze the
vehement necessities of delivery. What are these?
– I will tell you – they are being timely, and having
a hold. These things drive the acclimatisation of
sitting on chairs of wonder.


A good piece of the puzzle relays its position, and
we find something better to rest our eyes upon.

And then, like a scramble in the ointment, things believe they can be done. Do not be stationary in this part of the world. We must pay attention- Yes.


Having the sort of adventure that we are talking about. There is a life line to savour, and something to guide all ships. We run, and the mischievous come. What a sight for the eyes of lore. I drink water here, only because I can.


Coming close to the edge, but not going over. Being nice to neighbours, and having a challenge given. We send our teleology through our sense of it, and have as a feeling much to deride. I think of you these past weeks – there can be nothing more.


A count, and what is insoluble. A quick walk, and then the night. I love this more than ever, but what is in tandem, cannot be shown. What follows, holds the daylight in check. There is now a well-spring, one that doesn't fall away.


Treasuring the soul of it – we glide in forums like a new found heart. There is a chance we will tether our motion to the sea, and then give the land a satisfying embrace. Come now, we are the weather of it. We are that which has the feather.

The vicissitudes of life. We encounter them, and have as the brick and the cable more than is enough. We transform, in the movement up and across, there is what we need. Things come – good things, and our lives improve.


The coastline knows the sense of it. The coastline knows more than is tread upon. I have as the mirror and the sand, a little piece of the dried and stable. It comes it wells of fortune and place. The things we must do, are the things that are arranged.


Forests do not plunder. Forests only wait for their chosen ablutions. Come now, there is a suffering without surmise, and it is here that the tension diminishes. I look on, and know that the well is deep, and has much water – we must drink.


A harrowing need to send a letter. It comes, and then goes, and then finds the latch through which we climb. There is now a falsetto amongst the embers of fate. It dries as much as it can, and wriggles in close. I will find no other way.


Jumping in, jumping through – making light of it, despite its depth. I seek no redress, and have as the song and the heart a favourite lullaby. Do not retract anything. It is first in thought that we have as shelter. There is a maze to be gotten.

## And for a Moment Everything Seemed Fine

A missing piece – what we hoped, has been achieved. What we love, is the time it takes. I listen closely, but am not one to gauge the temperance on a scale. There is a little know wayward abeyance that loves its own motion. Let it.

A sense of camaraderie – one that doesn't diminish. I have heard, that trails in the night sky have as their wish a solemn rite, one that arcs in temporal abandon. I have not seen the template force itself over trains of feeling down – at all.

The height we find at the behest of suffering, is more than we can even comprehend. What is not lost, is the further accompaniment. Some things sing, and some things deride, and all of it put together is now a pulse in a languished heat.

Gravitating, and seeing what is fresh. I love what we find when we look. I love the sights we have in time to the destination of heart. That much can salvage a crew. That much can see the awnings for what they are. We are here to stay.

There is nothing like this in all the world. There is nothing like this in the half of it. Shall I rasp? Shall I clasp? Shall we hall the tins of phantom entrees? There is like a new film that layers the old. Come now, do not believe in renegade harps.

A little piece of magic is all we need. A little piece of the case to sharpen our wits. And then, like a mistletoe you can't stand under, a shape emits. There is within me all that has come to pass. There is here more still.

What is left of the meal. There is a simple remedy, one that owns delight as much as it curtails the dawn. I have figured in times of disarray, that which cannot be tethered, is not the centrepiece, but the overarching frame. I long for the distance.

Begrudgingly, but without effort, the stall of it winds true. Never before have we sent our tasks to such a target. There is a concourse that delivers. There is a sense we have that cables know which way to turn. That is why we relate to all.

There is a happening that lauds the basis of the white – the colour that holds so much in its hand. There comes a space, in which is thrown the destiny of all that harbours. I think now of you, and all that you appraise. There can only be what is.

What is it that we seek? What is it that we tread upon? There is a Dias, that gives the heart we find new found strength. And then like a bolt of

## And for a Moment Everything Seemed Fine

lightning, there is a rest we wish we had never cajoled. This is what it is for. This is what erupts.


Giving a gracious hand. Giving what the numbness says. Being pleased, but not over-rated. Having what we need, but not closing in. Having what we need, but having the cycle of it. There is a nuisance in the middle – right here.


There is never a suffering we can't deal with, in some way. Suffering now, means much, later on. This is the form it takes. It takes much to move us away from it – and it can't stop. There is a pause to, a pause that gives us a ready turn.


What have we sought – but all that will come. What have we been inside of, but the trepidation of an age. There is a pleasure here, one that seeks in less of an urn, and more of the transpiring. Can there ever be more than this?


Hobbling, but still going. A form of height that does not relinquish. There is a weather here, one that gives what is true to the sage. There is nothing we can say about what occurs, but that the timbre of the vault sustains a delectable wonderment.


I hold you – not because I can, but because it is needed. I am one not to shy away from the fire. There is a light to be had, and something to see in harrowing times. A feeling we don't often have, is here to take us through.


A set of equations to help guide us. And here, where there is no noise, the whisperings of today, become the grandness of tomorrow. What is left of our ease? What is left of the way we had? What cautions the residual. There is much.


Passing the test, this much has its hand upon us. We linger – but not for too long. We are encased, but not perturbed. There comes a gumption that is not of this world. It has a directness, but nothing of what we are used to.


What is the vicissitude, but a journey from here to there, from there to elsewhere? I know of nothing greater, than to have our hand on fate, and shoo away the suffering of it all. We can do it – and we must. And we do – for our future.


To trust in things is what we must do. There is a heaviness that rinds as it seconds – that opens as it lies afar – that comes as it pleases, and knows when the moment is close. Come now, I frolic in the embers – I dance amongst the dew.


There is a voice we all have. When times are difficult, we all can resort to it. And here, where we stand tall, there is a burning bright that hurries as it senses the way. What we flounder around for, is nothing short of all. But this will keep it safe.


Vehement, and standing in. Nothing but what dins. Nothing but what sings. Come now, a sense that riles. A sense that cajoles. Something like the tapestry of light. The combined longing of forever. I arc, but do not see. I have, but do not find.


A vision, one that says, in a resounding sort of way, 'further', and then sinks in. There is now time to move, and time to see things straight. Do not invigorate the pile, it will not stand it. Be in the density of it, we will show what the climes say now.


What is a wisp, is nothing more. What is a tenacity, is simply that. We move, and in one circular motion, we lever the mandate of the people. Wring it true. Wring it live. We can only be when we want to be. We can only have what is not placed.


My luck is here to tangle. My art is here to find. And then, like a radar in the straights of it, we believe in something out of the ordinary. What is the clawing we seek? What is its form? What is its name? All these things come together. We should relay.

We suffer, but what is this but an anathema on reality. There is, deep inside, a trigger that combines all we go through, and assigns our reward accordingly. There is something else at the end of suffering. We will find it.


Having the steel to continue. Being all in. Being what we call the whimsical. And then, like a whining that doesn't last – here, oh, here, we have life, and love, and all the tears we can shed. This is the time for it – let us writhe.


Carrying on, without so much as a smile, or a whimper. Or in the middle of the journey, something that makes us hurry. Something that makes us new again. Something that harbours no ilk, nor milk to dry our wet hands.


What do we do? What do we say? What have we here? What have we there? These questions lead to answers. But what are the answers? This is the gist of it. We come, and there are things to do, and ovals to watch out for.


A mesmerising – one that doesn't stop. A fellowship of outlining places. A new encounter with the grasslands of the world. We hold our heads up, and see once again. Never in nature has there been so much.

Salubrious and with the measure of it. Time to embark, and say your will. There is always thought for this. There is always the well and the pipe. And like a rain that sets in, there is nothing more to it. Nothing more than the reason behind things.

We have encountered the blackness of an overarching configuration. And here, where the moisture of life awakens – merriment, and the hands of the district. We must not do less than is needed. It is here to wander and to rebuke.

Suffering – it has its use. It has more than that. It has the power to transform our lives, if we let it. An ancient art, the art of suffering. It is something that just comes to us, as naturally as that. It is in us to make it work for us.

Hanging a plant in a new home. Hanging a picture there to. There is a mansion at our disposal, a place that concurs with everybody, and seeks incredible displacement of the embers of things. Do not create an angle – it cannot.

And then like fading in due north, there is solidified a brochure of composures, one that eeks out life in places unknown, unseen. Come and be a part of the repertoire, you will see more than composure can give. That is fine, that is great.

Nestled in – like webs in a tray full of warmth. I
hear your volition – it concurs with the saying.
There is much we must endeavour to say and do.
There is much, that holds the place in twine and
around. Court the fence, and then the morrow.
You will dance.


Glad to be home. Glad to be still. I encounter
nothing less. Do not find your arbour here – or
rather do, but at your leisure. Come to the feeling
of the trident pool. There is an astounding array of
things. Do not repent. We simply love.


Gathering ourselves up for something special.
Gathering up the papers of past lives – this year I
did this, and this year I did that. I have as a sequel
to the show more of the training of things, rather
than the wool in the vision. I will eventuate.


The pain we often feel is the world's, as it picks us
up, and travels us around. We accept it, simply by
living. And then, with cognisance sharpened, we
move it to where it should be, that is improving
what we have, and giving it space to grow.


A host of garden beds, all in a row. There comes a
music not of this world. There comes a message
from the deep. There comes something new,
without the hinderance of things past. Without the
desperation to seek, and climb.

## And for a Moment Everything Seemed Fine

There is here much to curve through, and much to abandon. We laugh, and play, and hold the tension in our hands, and love the nonsense of it all. A great metallurgy comes, and fires in, and harps through. There will be a time.

I know of the web and the spire. Two important things. I know of the spire and the rice – two things unrivalled. Do not tally, a walk will do. I love this tundra, as a sacred land. I love all the show, and misbegotten revelries. What is here, is here for all of us.

What carries us? – What gives us heart? What lifts us, until rainbows have a partner? There is something in us that dreams in placatory wonder, and has as its willow the nuances of the tribe. Do not feel the way, we will requite.

And then, like a curb on the road, difference and sweet excess. I will gather things such that none can be wanted. And then, like a start from the beyond, more of a figure than not. I will come for the hedges to be shorn, and then lifted.

What has life given us, but a need to pounce? What are the seeds for, but everything that we can expect. There is a weathering that steels. There is a shying away, that hopes in time to be in league.

We will only show you what is written on the cards.


There courses through this life a need do away with suffering, and this is how we do it. Up and across. Height and then betterment. Full lives, this much is here. Can we feel the strenuous heart? Can we ennoble ourselves for the moment. Let us.


There is a fable at the centre. There is a ransom at the edges. Do not climb without ropes. And then, like a glad-fly we retrieve the signpost from the ardour of it. Is this the staple and the knave? Is this what has us so entranced? Let us see.


Drawings that make up a design – but a design for what? And here, when we least expect, a new direction, one that comes from the test of it. There is chanceless grace at our disposal. And in this, lies a gap. And in that gap is everything.


We hold on. But not for the reason you might expect. It is an air beneath our wings, one that says, in the first instance, 'hear' – and that we do. But there is more. We do not have a temper in the face of all that is. And so, we hold, and hold on.


Vestibules, and what we see. Vestibules to enter, and then relax through. A servicing that allows for the kind of thing that never accompanies. I will walk – exactly a mile. In this time, the world turns, and has as its trajectory all of us combined.


There is no difference between the wind and the sorrow of it. We reach, but what do we reach for? We let ourselves be, but for what purpose? There is nothing left. On the contrary, we have everything before us – such is the way of it.


A blissful slumber – one that talks itself to sleep. I wonder, as it were, whether this is a time of rest, or one of action? Is the freight we haul going to lever the night in its pulse, or will we never have all that is for pasture?


Discomfort – there is a remedy for this – it is the future that we see. The future and all that will be. Come now, do not respite – but let your banner unfurl. There will be something in the midst of it to argue for, and to sublimate.


A horseradish, one which doesn't come all the way home. A vying for position. A hope that we can stand. There is a placement of cold things on hot things – which will be vanquished? A litter not strewn. A heart not beating. We will fly.


A gift given in motion – a gift given in repose. I argue with the pulse of it - and know that ease is not what we are about. We tackle, and see the score. We obviate, and draw that line in the sand. There will be tendrils to gather.

What is this for? What is this to do with? The load is light, but what of the drama? There can only be this. There is always this. And then, like a fable in suites of tenacity, there is a reality that must be cautioned. Be one to be still.

Fibre, fibre of the soul. We lurch, and are seen to be parted. We fire, or have it, to keep us warm. There is a miserly mode, that hankers distance more than is ready. What of it, is the speech. What of it, is the perfunctory.

A chain that can break if we want it. A change in the gut – one of strength. And now, without recourse, we wander – on legs of sheer readiness. I will not have the rest. I will not have the time to say, 'Hey, hey'. Do not be precluded.

There is never enough time – time to do things we need. There is a blast from the pedestal, one that closes in on fate. And now, without the newness of it, we climb that bit higher, and know that things will be in the offing.

Catching the density of it. Being appalled at the closure. Mistaking the rise for the plateau. We take our chances, and see the headlights far off in the distance. Is this where we lay? Is this the troubling key that holds the show? We will see.


Ranging on out, we come to that difficulty that is suffering. What do we do now? We wait – we experience – we heighten - we transform. This is the source of it. Then we direct, how would we like our lives to be? It is that simple.


Moistening the dryness of it. Holding the rainbow in our hands. Being one to trickle down. There can always be something to rival this. But what of the merriment in the stalls? What does it say to the dawn, except, 'what a tragedy it could have been'.


Giving up so much, so much, and then taken life by the scruff, and just proceeding. That is the way to move. And then, like a settled piece of chamber, we echo all the shadows that ever engaged. We must find a way, and we will.


There comes a time to pattern, and one to frolic in the sun. I like what it is I see. I like what it is we have before us. There is a change in the wind of it. There is a mobility that is sought for. There is now a thing we must do. And we will do it.


Seizing the picture frame, and then hanging the print. There is something of the guile of it. There is a touch too much magic to decipher the reeds. I

have as a limit to this, all that strangeness can
give. A tired crescendo, and all that will pass.


A conscious remark – one written in the dark. A
fairly done by thing, one that rings true. A fairly
done by conundrum, one that highlights the
tapering – the tapering of this to that. We stand
mesmerised, very much before the seam of it.


I have heard it said, some suffering crushes. To
this I might say, we might bring forward the notion
of lives past this one. But this is up to people for
themselves to formulate. Sometimes it is good to
determine what is best for each on their own.


A well being that hurts. A tried and often remarked
nuance that hears the fence post before time. We
do not languish, not here, not anywhere. We clean
the settee, and have as a stock of it, more than
the dice and the throw. More of it.


A gracious smile – one that does not release in
wonder. Come and be a part of the grand
adventure of life. It is here we wander, for more
than the trope hurts. Come now, do not listen past
the ruck and the remorse. Please be nice.


A wanting that drives us. A wanting that cools
itself in times a levity, times of happiness. I see
you in the middle of it, and know that the sand will

not rise for it, not for now, nor ever. Is this what we find when we plunge? Is this what we find?


A madrigal that loosens the pall. A happenstance that believes in fate. I have no means to occupy the parts of this that have gone to the highlands for the repartee. Do not silence the land, it is up to us. Do not silence what it is that barks away.


A considerable applause that comes. A sense of belief that harbours anything we want. Here like a maestro, we do not hesitate to bring forward what is instantaneous in us, and then back again, through thick and thin.


Missed by an inch. Never curtailed – but by whom? I let the instructions fly, and then blast a feeling or two. There is a window or sorts, one that looks out onto the bay. From it, we can see forever, and all that will lay. From it.


The vicissitudes of life – we see their allotment, and their arrangement, and we gasp at the very sight. But what we must do is harness them, and bring them to bridle. In this, once done, we have succeeded. A new life beckons.


Holding the reigns, pushing back the tears. We single this out – we single out a myriad of vantage points, to be the pensive and the verse itself. I

know of no other smiling, despite recollections,
despite the call of all.


This is what we have now. This is what calls itself
by grandeur and by surmise. I am the one to figure
clearly and with much thought. There, in the tin,
there it waits. There it lingers. I will have it not
sown, to anything but the incandescent and the
road.


A higher arc, one that holds all that shall pass. Do
not spit venom at the vehemence of it. Do not
angle the dye this way. Do not have as a fortifying
notion that things will believe of themselves. There
is more to life, except the encore and the maze.


Running quickly, we thrive in the house upon
which we speak. There is a nothingness in the
middle, and here where the disjointed and the
jovial haunt, we catch a moment to see our breath
unfold, and see it more than ever.


A hunt for the daylight – we will find it still, and still
breathing. We open our eyes, and have the world
at our disposal. Do not find the congestion
wanting. There is a new type of holding that treads
a life. And here, something special – something
great.

Erasing the lead, and taking it on. Being precocious, and never being afraid. There is a temperature that excites. And in the meantime, something from the family occurs – something small and derisive, that rectifies itself almost immediately.

What more is this, this thing we call suffering? Anything can be transformed into anything. This much is how things go. Let us have a new life, a-blazoned with debris from the sharp of it. We must not look too much forwards. This much we see.

And there we have it. There we go. A long-lost bravado gets us the depth of it. There is a saying that reprises as it jumps in – "Look at all the people gathering – what are they doing?" And here where the mistress of the age comes back in, more of the suit.

What is it we know of? We know of noting in particular, except the tangent from here to there, from coast to coast, and ambiences in between. I have found something that is worth a gallon a go. Maybe as we inch, I will preclude.

And now, like a starling in the summer-time, a life that has hardly known air, we see her pass, and watch her journey. You can see for yourself of the difficulty of any journey. This one is resplendent. But what of the life of it. It will pass.

Come now, not as a vision in twos, or threes. But in fours and fives. This much comes as a winding passageway. We lift our ocean, and seek the chance to dive. But what is this, but being pallid? What do we digress with – more than is enough.

A trend in the banter of tales untold. A namesake that roars on. Come now do not catch a hold. Do not syphon the dry. Only give your all if you have it. We have no choice. There is a lack of a reaction. We will cross the path.

A wisdom that imparts - but imparts what? Imparts the rose and the thorn. The majesty, and the preposterous. We sing, but to what tune? We live, but for what purpose? There is a game to be had. One without the slightest nomenclature.

I ask you to gather the webs of a thousand spinnings, and have as your ally all that dust can bare. The choice is not of this desire, nor of this incendiary spark. I come to play, but what is the version we adhere to. We will fall into line.

What is the reaching we know of? What is its time and vertigo? What is the notion that is set in plaster thick as dominion. I have as the solid intransigence a sapping and a falling – a relaying and a sport. A coaching and a de-vicing.

# And for a Moment Everything Seemed Fine

How are we to do this? How can we transform what is painful into what we want? It is not up to us. We simply lead our lives and it happens. We encounter suffering everyday, and each day we move closer. Maybe not now – but in the future.

A clanging sound, one that doesn't dismiss. A restive placation of things un-blemished. There is a mouth piece, that all the world can here. And in this sound, we pick up what we need, and dreamily show our path to be true.

A foraging that ignites. A flash of light, and all that it contains. There is here something that gives no more of the parting wish, and more of cadence of the journey. Do not follow any quicker. There is breakfast to attend to.

Aggrieved, but not sorry. Tender, but not like the night. A silence that transfigures, and a chasm that envelopes. There is much here to do. There is much here to say. There is a heel on this foot that enjoys the walk. We will do so.

When we tag what the night will give – here, yes here, there hums a gale to the foremost parts. And when the most precious of those things has had its pass, there, oh there, we will see the sink hole for what it is worth. Enough to get out of.

Pain, and disbelief. We work at it no matter how long it takes. It is here, we find that catch that alleviates the storm, and ameliorates the weathering, much to our enjoyment. There can only be one way. And that is through.


A gusto that has nothing to send. And now, like a forbearance entrusted, we lap into shores untold – but it is as unmapped, that we seek what it is we need found. And then like a winter blast, there is much time to change the guard, and have it sent.


What was once fierce is now tempered. What was once enslaved is now free. And then like a riling off the fence, we sing the plaudits of our might and…away to the distance. What have I feared, but what will come. What have I known but all.


There is magic here, that rings and defies, and gives rest. I have the chance to once again flail at the light of the day, and see its tremendous curvature linger in steel over the blue. I have as the furthest que a wandering that believes itself capable.


Hope to the next in the series. Finding the darkness appealing. Being very much in lieu of the daunting. We call out our commitments, and know with deep knowing they are fine. And now, like soda in the summer, we tune our stars to the right pitch.


Having a near taste in the mouth. Having a science of heart to accompany the fjord. And then like a massaging, we embark once again on the nearest road, to again see what travelling can do. Is there more to partake? Let us see.


Judgement of the class of things. We follow, but to what end? We laugh, but from which strength? There is now a simplicity in the making of it. Up, down, and through. What we gathered is not so much an errand, as a lynchpin of thought and deed.


We must conquer our suffering, and we can do that by enjoying the natural fruits of what we are going through. There is time enough to settle the score. What suffering takes, we give back in our own way. There is a place for this. Let us be sure.


A future for the heart. A scientific recognition of the reality of what is. We fight, but for what understanding? We listen, but our hold is quick. We seek the sanguine, but enough of the hill of it. We locate the vine, and have no need of the simplicity of it.

What is fashioned is not of the accord. What is diligent cannot be here eventually. And then like a fire through the fog, we see ourselves descend from the height, giving much insistence to our efforts. There is something more we can give.

A watershed moment, in the curtailing of this to that and back again. I will not linger, nor wash away my tears. They will stay, and have as a dimension the rumblings of all that shall be and all that shall come to pass. We reckon another vantage.

Before we know it, a ship comes into harbour. And like the magicians of the solid ground, there comes a mighty embrace. Why do we seek that? What is the cause? What is the temper? Millenium, and all that is here to be offered.

Do not fill your shoes with august energies, the terrace is here to stay. We are on the way to a place of unrecognisable life and lore. Do not see the trees for what they are. We have as our countering a vociferous conclusion. It is said.

Catching the last of it – being ensnared by the mistress. I have as an ally my only font – with this I write. To be the simplest thing. To be that which only the waiter can bring. And now we love what it is that keeps us going – and then?

## And for a Moment Everything Seemed Fine

A deeply melded part to play. A type of thing that doesn't ring. Any more of the fibrous, and we will have to depart. Is this the way through, and forwards? Is this where temptation leads? I have never seen the day quite like this.

When you are hurt, just observe yourself. This is the heightening of consciousness, which is the first step towards the transformation of the possibility of improvement. Life exceeds expectations here. We can never come down.

A forest bed teeming with life. A sense we have that things will turn out right. And then, like a rose petal in the spring, there comes an amazing title to claim. In this we judge ourselves aright, and feel that the gesture is all in the sun – we will come.

A mission to accomplish the beleaguered and the sound. I hear your navigation that unlocks the box of freedom – that unhinges the bold and the lucky. Do not send yourself to sleep here – there is a need to unlock the gate and have it roar.

And then, with combined speech, we come from the town that knows no district, and the shore that has no sand. Be the one who reckons, reckons the irreconcilable. And then like a jar in the crux of it, we hold sway, and never look back.

A testament to the noise of it. A harsh way to sound the openness of it all. We come, and are taken. We smithy and see ourselves recover. And then, like a burden in flight, there is more to see, and more to engage. We will finish.

A cry in the night. Something to relish. Something to harp on. A regularity that forces a twinge. What is there, is not here. What is here is not there. We caution, and are told which direction. We listen, but always in threes.

It is like this – we sing to the highest point, and then come down to reach earth. But what is it we truly desire? What is it we have that can be chosen? There is a likeness that pertains to derivatives of the soul, and here we will not admonish a single one.

There are forms of suffering that are deeper than others. And which we receive depends on us. The deeper the suffering the greater the rewards. And here amongst the ruins, a new life, one that is transfigured from the old.

A long walk – one to dismiss anything we harbour as objective. Do not range in wild format. Because it is here that the wantings of fireflies achieve their most ardent passion. It is like this – we get up, we go, we stop and we go again. This is plain.

And now, like a wager that fills the nearest path, we come back down, and ledger the waste in a semblance of configuration. We are here to dispute nothing. And then, as a difference in height, we come for the sand, and rain on the fairy lights.

A sort of calm – the sort one would only feel once in a lifetime. It must be revelled in, and then remembered – where, and when. There is nothing to it. The seeds we carry are for the birds. They enjoy the companionship the most.

Having something of a time of it. There arcs back to infinitude all that must be done. But can the bluestone beautify the dark? There is a soul to chase, one that laughs at its own enlivening. We must be careful – the edge of things riles.

Whispering to who knows where. Feeling the pain, but continuing. Often times we seek shelter from the tempest, and this is what we find – we find love, and care, and compassion and all that suffices for the day. Do not simply be pleased, but that to.

There is a time for all that is here. There is a winding that stretches into the distance. I am reminded of a faraway place, one that is not yet here. And then, like the rainbow in the blue, a mesmerising effect, one that never leaves.

Unconscious, but breathing. We encounter our suffering like never before. We feel it – when will it go? But it comes again. When will it go? Finally, and without remorse it goes. We are left alone. The future will be ours. It is in the making.

A firelight that has never burnt, it sheds light, still (somehow), and knows that each passing day is precious, and the majesty of delivery hangs close. There is a new type of defence we practice. It is here, before our unbelieving eyes.

And then, like a wind that has no friction – there is more than igloos can embark without. And like a semblance in rain, there issues a new found desire, one that has as it skirting board the nearness of a major petal. Do not enrage.

A mighty jingle, one that laughs itself to sleep. I find what is closest, and then furthest, and then I shout for the native grind. Do not belittle the sun, it has no time to invigorate the chains that bind. Do this, and what will be will tarry.

Gaining speed, the top most portion has as its silk the differences in opinion that evoke. And then, like a sense unknown, there comes a beauty that accords faith, that drives the unhindered, to spacious exigencies that do not bite.

Withstanding – coming across. There are dimensions to this journey that have as their kind a warbling call. Never delimit yourself. Never once has the scene been trebled, nor excavated through. Just sit on your position, and laugh when given.

I see a place worth a solace, and a bark made to order. It is here I hunch, and here I stark. Never one to see the train, only hear its belatedness – I gather, and sing like a pool of chains delivered. What is the likeness of it? Expunged.

The pain of it subsides – what now? We wait, live our lives, and see things gradually accumulate. There maybe more suffering, and again we rise, and again we live and wait. The cycle comes and goes – but we accumulate. And there it goes.

The sea – the rush. The wind. What is next? Over and under. Committed to the hinderance. A stark reminder of the song of us. Never have we seen this before. Never has the waste been so recondite. I will listen for the gate.

A source for the kaleidoscope. Holding the arch back. Being concerned to approach. There is here the well-being of an age, but that is of no consequence but of the charge and the obstacle. This is what gives us our flight.


There is nothing more satisfying than a pose embossed. There is like something than cannot veer. And here, where the noise of life can never diminish, there comes a thought in each of us that can never stay. But we will capture it, before too long.


And now, insistent, we commence. There is a harbour for ships about to sail. It is a magical place, one that is steeped in lore and versions. We love this as we encounter. We love this as we slip and sweep, and carry forward.


Letting loose the tethers that bind. Having as a signal all that can never capitulate. We gather ourselves, but not for tomorrow. We gather ourselves, and only for the moment. We sing, but never for the crowd. We will be entrenched.


Let your discomfort fill you, there is a new horizon ahead. There is a taming that shows no sound of a backstep. What we thought would never come, has come. What we thought would never be, has become. Let us rejoice.

## And for a Moment Everything Seemed Fine

The steps we take now, are the steps that have made us feel lightheaded. The charm we bring with us, is that which will follow us. What is it we bring? What is it we turn? What is it that we cannot forsake? We will learn.

An amazing eventuality – we sit, and see more of the time that is left to us. There comes a friction in the wind. There comes a noise from the attic that is unfamiliar yet comforting. We see ourselves through glass eyes.

A faith in the tapestry of it all. I find myself aloof, but needing to find more. There is a displacement the stars feel, that we must not trade for anything or anyone. And then, instead of a noise, there is a sound. Instead of motion, there is a stillness.

Having the best focus for the charm of it. Knowing what is invigorated and left as insight. We feel the love of it plainly – we are told what it is before acceptances. But that is to say, we will not march to any orders, orders at all.

A furthering that musters. A new privilege that does not curtail. We will bend the sail in two, before we are through. There makes a rounding order, one that cannot sleep through. I will envisage what comes next – it is time.

There is a space, between every breath of the wind. In this space is something that surprises. It is a gap that is filled with memories. Each memory makes a sound. All we must do is listen, and lo they are found. Hear the past.

There is a motion that does not stop. Here, where suffering meets the mind, sparks and things that are shaped ethereally. There is no time to stop. We must move in such a fashion as to secure our reward. Suffering and its transformation.

Accustomed to the shore, there lingers a new need to see what life has in store. There is here something that should always be reckoned, reckoned and then released. There are countless things to pass in the night.

Having to secure life from the daylight, there is a hunting that doesn't injure. There is now a tom foolery, that lags behind the rest. And here, where the silence of the fashioning commits, there harks a new fathoming. One that doesn't understand.

A vacuous appraisal – one that senses the right way to go. I see you now, walking through the thoroughfare, and like a farther seeking, there washes the nighttime embrace, like the sound of it never was. We hurtle, but to what effect?

And then, like a shiver, the melting we dream of only gets stronger and stronger – until – abeyance and all that is clear. I look edgewise, and see the temple glistening in all manner of display. There is a troop here, we must entreat a path.

A random adventuring – we should be more able to the task. And then, like a rise in the test, we fall like spectres of belief never once arguing for ourselves. And then like a wisdom that has come for the dance – a beguiling – one that simplifies.

Wrangling with the dice – we see all. We see all, and never let go. A signpost to the tutelage, and all that is remiss. Never once cry your name. Never once be indebted. There is too much to understand. There is too much.

A sight we see along the way. A desire that renders itself wholesome. Come now, the sleet and remorse are enough open our eyes afresh. I know of no other way. This way is the blindside to the territory. This much comes.

All we can do is harness what we are going through. And then take solace in the fact that things get better from here – our consciousness heightens, and improvement begins. What can there be other than this?

Whispering – like an attack of sunlight on the vision of things. Where are we most likely to go? Where is that which we most abhor? – Wrap it up, and send it through. Come now, the distance never really matters. I will not abandon.


A hot intensity leaves us lounging. A new way to be beckons. There is like something we have never seen. A truth-scape, that harbours all. Do not relinquish fate – it has come to stall. Do not be the one to be still. That much is a cacophony.


And then, like writing on the clouds, something special. I find what it is that keeps us going. I wrap it up, and then see myself diminishing. Much faith, and much innocuous lemon arranging. There is time past the hour.


A figure of speech – one that never leaves. There is now considerable allotment to be had. I see your back, and know you to be a ghost of vast complexion. I sense there is nothing else. But what of this? We wrestle in, and never leave.


Which way is left? Which way is straight? Questions – let us answer them. In fact, no let us guard against them. There is a tremendous willing here. A tremendous about face. I love what we see here. There is a simplicity that doesn't waste.

What lot do we take with us? There is a breathing we do to accomplish. And then, like a stoicism we can handle, there looks onto the floor a sort of eagerness to accompany. But here, there is something we cannot contain. It is there.


Pain, and the level. We see ourselves again, and know that what we feel will not last, and that when things go, they go for us. And when things go, all that is left is what we want. This has evolved from thousands of years of humans encountering suffering.


A magic, not to be curtailed – not to be dismissed – not ever. And then, like a rogue element, we see the path ahead, and know it to be a stampede. But we are more than dreaming. In actual fact we surpass even ourselves. What is more?


A nice way to proceed. A nice way to carry along. And then, instead of the harness, we have the shooting across. Something we have not seen before. Bare witness to the temerity of it. Serenity burdens, and then releases. It is true.


A clown regard, one that dismisses as it breaches. One that entwines as it dispenses. Come and be the sharpness of the wit. Come and be the temptation and the sorrow. There is no foundry like this - no place to be ensnared again.

Holding onto fate – we know that what we see won't entreat. What we hear won't embark – and then like a level of success, there re-engages the dismal and the fray – that is the way. We love what we are, we love what we contest – Yes.


Watching, feeling, using things to their optimum. I sense a change, but what is it? Is it the brass off cables of tumult? – Is it the sound of marshes, entrenched in light? Is it the willow we hear – a sound that continues to march? We will find.


There are times we wish we could hide – but the world has no escape. In our suffering we catch the last of the somnolence and sheer it away. We arrange our life in preparation for change – change of the utmost care. There is wear.


I know that in the fence is a dreaming. And here, where the mast does not beckon, there is a small amount of calm to be had. We know it to be clear of all that can tarnish. The mystery of the fellow traveller, is just that – here we will find.


A condolence that sings. An embrace that seeks itself in the trellis and has as a balm the mightiest of things. Do not repress that hail – it will come any way. I see you shout, from the top of it. I see you listening, from the deep. I see you.

## And for a Moment Everything Seemed Fine

Almost crawling, the legs are for this road alone. I come, once again, in fields of darkness, fields of sight. I sense the mining will come together with the fruit. I am of the plangent, and the silver. Be prepared – light is amongst us.


Be insistent as to what you want – your suffering will take you there. And then, like a radish field peeled with life, there comes a new way to see. A new way to envelope. And a new way to delineate. Watch for the breaches – they bite upon arrival.


There is now a sense we have that the tower is here for the raging. Without circumference nor letter, we hear what we must. It will be as a side-shift in perception that culls the mind, and inserts a generous spirit in all that is. It will be done.


Mischief – and exuberance. We play, and seem to know which way we are going. We play, and see the sempiternal emerge. 'What is this?' I hear you cry to the daylight, and seemingly find your place. There is more than the dawn can take.


Mind your step – These journeys don't tarry. We must forgive the past; it is all we can do. We must delve deep if we are to survive. And here where the sand of it doesn't give an inch, there, oh there, a mighty composure transcends.

We sublimate our suffering, and choose which way it will turn. But it always goes up - up and across. The across is what interests us here. This is where the new life turns. See what we can do with this. It will come again.

What are we to do now? What is the lounge, and the perfunctory? There comes a passion to be present – present to all who have come. There is like a ragged hill that does not see itself in grandeur, nor in tiles. This much commends the keepsake.

We saw a play last night – superb. We saw a newness emerge that doesn't reminisce. I hear of the triangle and the missive, and the time that will pass. I know that the juncture is here for the smart and the rude. We will excavate the scene.

What more can we do? What more can we say? What more does the semblance of the horizon have? I arch, and am ready. I feel and see the tempest run for me. I love what it is that keeps the ball in motion. There is a libertine to be.

Fishing for it. Giving life, life where it is due. We cannot savour more of the sound – but that is okay, okay for the rest of us. Do not signal the break of day, it comes only to have a harrowing at our expense. This much cannot be done – but still.

# And for a Moment Everything Seemed Fine

Stillness, and the breeze. Aforementioned and acclimatised. I see of nothing else. But here, here we joust. Never saying when. Always distant and afar. I catch on something of proportion, and let the merriment commence. This much.

What we have turned is something that has no holes. It is something we grimace at initially, but then come to admire. The section of the recipe we are reading defies description. This is as it should be, for fun and merriment. I will chase.

What is suffering anyway? It causes us pain and distress, this much is clear. But what of the rest of it? What does it do? It interferes, and slows us. But that doesn't have to be the case anymore. We can use it to our advantage. That we will do.

Rushing in, and rushing about. There is something about the time of it that we find appealing. But what is that? It is the flavour of it, if that makes sense. The taste of time. We linger now, and say to ourselves we will never acquiesce.

Come now, be beautiful – be beautiful in a garden of the beautiful. I think of a butterfly that flies unknowing of its own beauty, and the pleasure it gives. This much is where we should stand. In amongst the ruins of an ancient castle.

A touching sentence that unfolds as it uplifts.
There is a time spent that harbours no ill. No ill,
nor keepsake. I render things first and foremost in
twine, then in silk, then in paper, then on canvas,
then in marble. This suffices for the arc of things.


Much that we want to see. Much that has as its
dimensions all the girth of the world. Much that
transcends the able and the rind. Do not hesitate,
the wheel that turns, turns for us. We sing, but
where are we going. It will tell.


And now, like never before, we stand to attention,
and blazon our name on all the faults at sea. I
catch myself, before I fall, and know a rendition of
something that has heart as its length, and a great
grandness as the apogee of all things.


Very similar to the last. Very similar, in the tray.
We guide ourselves with two things to cope with.
And that is the tarnish, and the velvet. I sense
your dis-ease, but what have I got that is not the
harbour and the well-spring.


Sublimation – this is the key. We take what is
dross, and turn it into gold. And that gold is our
lives post our suffering. But yes, of course there
might be suffering then to. But we are at liberty to
sublimate that to. And then the future, utmost.

## And for a Moment Everything Seemed Fine

We have as a companion through these journeys - the night. The night as it goes. But what of the rest? We have as a centre-piece the distant stars, stars that make our own journey seem small. And there we exist, in the smallness of it all.

I am on the road of it. I see my way through. Do not encase the tether nor the bond. Do not entreaty that sound we make when we go to bed at night – it is the same sound that the trees makes. I sense all and have not the disposition to fly.

And now, without the time of fashioning and the world, there believes another sensation – one that is in the wind of all. I lie down, so that I can hear more clearly, and in doing so I open up ways of being and ways of stretching that only flint.

What here does not diminish? What here comes in pace? There is nothing like the air of it to send us trudging through the snow and into oblivion. We come once again to our senses, and construct a new life from the old. That much is possible.

Hankering for the flood. Doing what it takes. We linger, but only for the good. And beside it all is the transit – a thing that can never holds us back. We walk in circles, but never to destiny. I listen, but only because I can.


An off the cuff speech. One that bends. And then, like a fabulous departure, we gather ourselves once again to see how far we can go. It is here we sit, once more, to see the space at our disposal. Catching the tape, and turning it around.


When does suffering start? It has had no starting point. When will it end? It ends with us, and our commitment to see it finish. Even if we don't see the end of it, we can improve things to the extent they are manageable.


A harbour in a sea that has no despair. We look to the west. We look to the east. We look to the north. We look to the south. And here it goes – over hand and foot we search, and in this search is all that is precious. We will not stop.


Covering the hills – we glimpse that which is most important. We see our lives that cost nothing but the air we breathe. There is a ransom on the skill we have at life. There is now a swanning that gives way to the preciousness of it all.


A future bearing that gives us the tendency to believe in things again. And now, like a causeway in the gloom, we find our feet, and never once think to cast a lonely stone. There is a hike to be had, around the salt of it, which we know and savour.


Holding the day aloft, we catch what is easiest first, and then move down to the hardest. We are still there at the end of acceptances. Do not be privileged – it is unknown to be short here. There is everything we need, right here.


There will never be a place for this. There can never be what the hold out says. And now, like a fold out address, the template of the falling mass envelopes all that is. Come and be a part of the grand show. It will not hurt.


A mastery of the hills. A test of strength. What we are given, is nothing short of the tributary. And like a fog in the middle of winter, we sail forwards and through. Never one to engage in the sweep and the tarry, we ride like never before.


Pain and discomfort – what are they anyway? By the time they are finished, we have a new life, one that doesn't look back. It is here we find our strength, and know it to be worthy of us. There is a semblance of calm that comes.


Sorting out, being with, and being-without. And new need, one that harbours all that is. Do not sense the stream, it is for the morrow. Do not reconcile the detritus, it has as its dimension all that we can give. There is a part here – we will wonder.


Gaining in passion, this is where we live. Gaining in knowledge, we have nothing else to give. There is a festive clue, one earmarked for recovery. There is now a rectilinear motion, directed away from us. Its respite is given in twos and threes.


Forgoing, and not forerunning, there is a now a little distraction from the side-roads. And in this we develop ourselves, and are in congress of the meeting. Whether we will, or whether we won't, this much is decided. Come and be.


Foraging, and being perceptible. Wringing true, and never flighty. There is a load too hard to carry – but we will carry it – simply because it is too hard in itself. But what is this, something that diminishes as it encroaches? We will find out.


Considering the options – we turn to this. What it is, we do not know. What it is, we cannot say. And then, like a thoroughbred through the undergrowth, a science to it all. Like new things to do, and not for a moment. Like the balletomane.

## And for a Moment Everything Seemed Fine

Consideration of the form of it. A close relationship. Something that never smothers the embers. A catch in the cry. A long way away. We part, but for how long? Never before seen. A shield of wind. Something that doesn't partake.


There is something special about our life after suffering. It all comes together. But it might not last forever, so we must accustom ourselves to it being ongoing. But once we have grasped the movement, there is no stopping.


A ghost. There in the corner. Tingles up our spine. Do you believe? Do you believe in the nascent and the solid? There is here a chance to breathe, breathe a new breath. And then, like a whisper – new found longing and a conscious start.


The further we go – the further we get. The further we search – the further we find. And here, where the worst of it is in the reckoning, a joy to behold. Once and for all, we come. Once and for all, we say. Do not register our remarks. They will spill.


And now, the in-between of desire and its fjord. What we guess, is not of the sanctity, nor of the nuisance. What we guess, is of tale of it. And here, incessantly, and without care, there remains a trail in the dust. For how long it takes.

A crisis that passes. A silence that rings. What we thought was jasmine, is now a piece of clover. I hear what is said, but I cannot respond. It is unlike me to finish another's sentence. There can only be the wishing that abjures the sign. Yes.


There is might, and the desire for privilege. And when we come to the impasse of the soul, there resides a reaching, and a giving forwards, and all that doesn't hurt. Do we question ourselves? This is a later blind. We enter – but who hears the news.


A limping across, that harks no intrusion. We harvest what it is we need. And then, like a particle prepared in pure faith, there is something we rarely understand. Never before has the rice been so lovely. Never before.


What is anguish, and can it fight itself into oblivion? We can help it by letting our natural tendencies take over – up and across – and away it goes. There is a sleeping that takes shape, and suffering subsides for a moment – then life.


And then, like vapour through the sky, we set ourselves for the solace of it. It is not inclement either. I offer my hand as a token, and sail through the abyss like a wanting that never was. Do not dismiss the aegis of the play. It will come.

## And for a Moment Everything Seemed Fine

What is this we see? What is this we have? Two questions – one answer – the sea. Enough of the folklore, it has wrung itself enough on parting ways. Ways that shine, and become gilded. Ways that come un-announced, and are set there-in.

There comes a tiger, one that has not been here before. It lingers, like a feather on the air. Do not remind us what life is worth. It is a sanctioning that levies a disruption to the hall of it. I find you well. What of that? There remains a simulacrum.

Trying to budge the servitude is not something we can do. And then like a wall of courage, we come forth, and sharpen our heals on the listening of the harbour and the train. Do not despise us, we are simply here.

Withstanding – relaying. We chortle, because things seem fine. We hold, and then banish. We love, but only what hurts. We feel, like a ranger in the meadow. We laugh, because it is the thing to do.

A vision – it is prepared. A motion – one that carries all. I see you. I see you from here. And when it is gathered, the holding the sky does is like a famished colossus. Bored and yet still. I find the place to look, and it is not here.

Heart ache, are you listening? Come, you are no longer feared. You spill from your vantage – you spill what we need and want in our future. This much is a fortunate clasp. We transform you, and never look back. We have now what we need.

A start – a piece of the wind. I do not relinquish, nor try to encode. There is a triangle at stake, one that never envisages. I am calm, I cater, and then burrow. This is what happens to the crowd. Be of the morrow, and temptation will not arise.

A fairy tale to the start of things. A nice piece to be landed upon. There is here a path to follow, if you will. There is no snaking under the grass, nor being in harm's way. There is a willow that does not bend. There is a compassion that listens.

Voicing, and being hopeful. An insistence, that boils down into, and then away. I sense your conviction, and raise you a smile. There is an awkwardness in the middle of this room. And then a moment later it is gone. Fortune persists.

We hold hands, only because the raffish and the charm has as its hold on the night a vast expanse – one that is not of this world to see. I love what we have, but it gets better – we suffer and it gets better.

## And for a Moment Everything Seemed Fine

Twilight, and forgiveness. A worthy sense of wrong. Dilapidated, but sincere. Mesmerising, and in tune. A favour that has been asked. A sort of rounding. More that is hoped. A terrible scene – one that is soon rectified.

We wait, and all that will come has come. And then, like sawdust in keeping with its surrounds, we settle, and transpose the evergreens. There is a likeminded insistence, one that has as its barrier the triumph of the nettle. We will sort.

Suffering – it can come, at any moment. But we are ready. And we see it, we let it work. And then we spill – spill life's riches. There can be no going back. Poets of the ages have all known this fact, and pieced their work into it.

A silence that doesn't blend – and one that does. A noontide that envelopes us in beauty. A sense of what is there, and what is now. A servitude to life. A need to start again. Something that rebels, but not in earnest. What is here and now.

And now, we sense an important juncture. What is it we need to continue? What is it that we need to displace? These questions are not easy to answer. We need what we have, and that only. We need nothing more but to be sure.

Consigning the tapestry to history. We fly in the face of it. We mosey on through, and out, and around. There is a step we cannot take. There is a breeze we must avoid. And then, as snow in the desert, we persist, and lunge at the sun.


Fulfilling our destiny. Each comes to pass. Each has a say. Each portrays the wind in their own way. We do not catch the lullaby. We do not have the keepsakes of our own choosing. We let the ruffians loose, only to remind ourselves later.


Giving leeway, and then sending off. We travel, but for what purpose? We ring the bell, but the house is empty. We say our farewells, but to whom? There is something we shouldn't miss, but do. The effervescence of here is palpable.


A great store of heart. There is more than the trumpet here. There is a way with things. I am on the vessel, I cannot look back. I play my cards, and see the sight of it. There is a chance like no other. There is the time it takes. That is all.


Pain – it comes in many forms. Imagine if it was a gateway to something greater. A new start, a new beginning, one that trailed off into the distance. We can live that dream if we like. We can live it, and never sacrifice.

## And for a Moment Everything Seemed Fine

We are late, but the celebrations started early. We know our place, but this is an opportunity to have ourselves rise, and then, respite. The mission here is take a hold of life, and baton the numbness across, and never say when.

A charge forward, and then the dice. We encounter nothing more of the wheel, nor the dimensions of it. We ring our hands, and what is left, but the simplicity of it all. We build, from the stock, and then let ourselves go, with much to tell of.

And then like ice on a very cold day, we find our home, and settle in, for the wonder of it all. Do not part – there is a chamber afoot. Much regard for the levellers – they are here to see. And that they do. Come and see the window pane – it contorts.

A feeling we once had – a feeling that never returned. That much is known, but what of that which is left? We welcome the starlight, that has as its function the mystery of the tenacity in check. I will be still. Now that I know the time and its inclination.

Tiptoeing through and beyond. We argue amongst ourselves, that the measure of things is in the willows. Do not fret here, we test, and are tested.

We hear our song, and give a little more. The rains come. We see them approaching.


The nest full of the young. There can be nothing more, and nothing less. We cope with bandages on. And when we hear the cry to believe in solemn rites – rites of passage, there will always be enough said. Enough said.


The need we have to cast off suffering is a noble one. We can never get rid of it, but we can reduce its impact on our lives, and yes, enjoy the fruits of its transformation. Between its encounter, and its conversion in lives towards happiness.


What is there left, but the stars in the sky? What is left, but the motion of all that is? We wander, but through what? We linger, but for what timing? I see you now, like an arrow in the darkness. I see us, as we travel once again. Do not dissipate.


Conscious of the speed of it. A sound that doesn't belittle. We evoke, but for which endeavour? The time it takes is above us – and there it should stay. The time it takes is nothing like we were told. So here we are. Right in the middle.


Thriving, but for which space? Delivering, but on time – or late? We have as a fortress a construction that remains intact. There is a caution

in the trees that knows no bounds. And here,
where life begins again, something more to say.


Wrestling with what is left. Wrestling with the
staunchest of allies. We come, and are needed.
We envisage, and explain. There is more to do
here – more than before. And then, like Samson,
we couch, and come to the right conclusion.


All the guile we can muster. All the fanciful. All that
is real. All that transposes. All that we need. And
then, like a breaker in use, we saddle up the
notion of here to there, and with one flick, we
sense a new beginning.


A constant that unyields. Something we never saw
coming. What is that? Made for the roadside,
made for the debris. I come, but never linger. I
say, and am want to begin. There is an ounce of
energy left – we will use it to our advantage.


Causing something like a tendency from birth. A
sound we saw coming. A fathoming that links –
links in all manner of ways. We are still – only
because we can be. There is not the slightest
thing that can even be placated. Here we swing.


Angst – we hear it, we see it – it follows us. But
when it has us, we can fight back. Up and across.
Height. And then the improvement that comes. We

need not wait – whenever we suffer, we can convert, and in doing so win.


There is a new dimension to life. It is here, where we travel through the mist and rain, and all that ever will be. I will not slavishly attend, attend to the whereabouts of yore. We must listen, to where things are at their finest, here we will be found.


Finding the stone of it. Something with gravitas. We have ached for this moment. But what of the will, and all that will come. What of the silence, the silence that beckons. We try, and hold on, hold on to the mystery of it. There is now more time than ever.


Retrieving the play of it. Much to say, much to do. There is a windswept alley with nothing in it. There is a house, completely empty, with more of the same in the yard. Please sit. There is a motion to embark upon. We will see.


There is a seething that vanishes. There is a believing that evolves. And when we harbour the nearest fray, we come close to the end point of thoroughness. Be the window, and the wind will thank you. It is written, and is veiled.


A communication in verse. It starts with a reminder – a reminder of what is and what is not. And here, where the vision is thick, and the trancing doubles as a show, there comes a nuance – one that does not, in anyway, remind the players of their birth.


Pain comes in many forms. It is here we need to salvage something – and that we do, in the strongest way. Our consciousness heightens, we transform, and what we need comes about – in shorter or longer time. Come and see.


There was once a forest, one that drank of the dew in morning repose. And here, where we believe in the sorrow for what it is worth, there comes a founding bridge, one that splinters and buckles all the way to the mast. This is where it goes.


A seismic shift in the way of it. We are not prolonged here anymore. We laugh, and say, and believe and have as our soldering all the joy of incumbency. Do not dream of the place we are at – or maybe do. Come and be a sailor in a sailor's world.


What there is now is the tempest and the rile. We long for the keel of it. Come now, do only what you wish. We have never seen the board on the tray of it. Do not resist the temptation. Only revel in what you see. There can be no other way.

Friendliness, and all that transpires. We dash the might we have on the rocks of the intrepid. This is what we seek, and what we have always sought. There is a goading to the right of things, but not to the left. We hurry, and look ourselves over.


There, in the distance – there – do you see it? Does it dance for you? Does it invigorate the soul and body? We treasure these moments all too well. Come now, we see the twilight in shades of colour unknown. Here we will stay.


There is a feeling we once had, that has not returned. But that does not display the future nor tempest in sync. We come for the register, and stay for the lark. I have as a calling all the wild. All the while, sleeping, and stationary comforts.


What must we do to sublimate? Just be aware. It is a natural reaction to an unusual situation. We pass the trailings to the wind, and have as our recourse a summer of enlivenment, one that upholds the spirit of times. Give more like the rest.


Coming and going, never seeing. We set ourselves for the journey, and then commence. It is like we never came across the forest at all. I hear the way you idle, and know that in the middle, there is a commiseration that does not trigger.

## And for a Moment Everything Seemed Fine

What is more than this? What is more than the wiling through the density of the plain? We have as a shirt confidence in the conquest. I have the need to squabble past, and have as my vector the humbleness of the day. Be one to sail.

Four and two, squared. Like a raiment through the heart (and back again). I see the torn our wear of the bombastic, and see it float in dishevelment. I do not anger at the corset, nor take bondage at the wearing. We love to dispute, and so on we go.

A free lime juice, one that does not acclimatise to the morsels around. There is a sending and a receiving that throws off the cartilage around the ends. This more suits than the roughage around the tutelage that brings in rain, more and more.

A tremendous aversion – one that sulks still. I have as the trumpet the need to live truly. I have as the trumpet the desire to fulfill. There is a majesty in the workings of it. There is a fire in the surrounds of it. I wince, but only because I can.

A making that hauls the light. A making that says yes, we are worth it. I come for the difference between me and you, and know that the silence in-between is not for the clay, but for the basin. We love, but not for the skill of it.

There is a suffering that keys in deeply to who we are. It is something evolutionary in us as a species to respond. We encounter it, and then we have the capacity to manifest a range of thigs in life – a partner, a car, a house. We just manifest.

Gleaming in the noon sun, we hold ourselves close, and know that the challenge is before us. We come in mighty shades, like a glass on the fabric of salutation. There is a magic-like appearance, one that we have been prepared for. Never give in.

Something intangible about the journey. Something never tolling about it to. I hope that there is a whiling, one that arches as it sees. I love the tempest – it gives me what I want. And then like a tragedy written in several verses, we applaud at the end.

A much-needed boost, we are here to revel. We are here to revel, and here to co-value. There is so much we must cajole, and so much we must never witness. I love what it is that keeps the register flowing – and then towards the blue-green.

Fixing a direction, there is a nightly flight to different parts of this world – parts we don't see. I love the realm, but pity the stasis. It is like something that has rarely come, perhaps once or twice an age. There is a pool of sweat that beats - it will.

Distillation of the heart. A ransom note that is badly written. A stasis that becomes us. A little-known fact. A hard to come by figurine. Something that bedazzles. A charm that re-invigorates. We will always continue here. We will always inch forwards.

And now, in the spring, when the dance is of the marrow, and the wincing dices it up into sleeves, we order great reams of things – great reams of tarnish. And in this, we cover ourselves in soot, and burgundy aplomb. So much now for the consolation.

I see in the arduous and the found, large changes of the silk and torn umbrage. There can only be the twine that binds – the stillness that obviates – the crescent that turns. There is a fear that cannot be absolved. But look here – it is gone.

The suffering we encounter is impermanent, but the reward it gives us is great indeed. We just have to let our natural inclinations take over. It doesn't have to be a conscious act – it is an evolutionary reflex that does the transformation.

And like leaves in a market-place we are blown here and there, never to stop with a fumbling of this too that, but always to have recourse to answers as they are needed. I hear what it is that you say, and come back with buoyancy and charm.


A tendency towards configuration. A leniency towards what is scouring, and the mesmerising of the line. We encounter nothing other than what enlivens – but does it enliven us? A question to be answered in halves, and halves-with.


A luck-defying procedure, one that gives heart as it gives salt. I wonder – do we stamp our feet at the breaking of breath, or do we let the soil of it be a receptacle for new growth, new wonders. New letters, let us have them.


Much in abundance – much to be sure of. There is a kindness in the breeze at times. It is hard to believe the same breeze can turn into a gale, and wreak itself upon unsuspecting parts of the world. There is now a safety net.


More than that which is willing. We harbour our niche, and let go of the temporal, only to find the spatial is in our reach. I know of the pointing from here to there, it has a slowness to it that does not abscond. Treasure it, we will need it.

And now we walk – very slowly at first, then faster, and then as a crescendo, faster still – but we are still walking after all. There is something that lets the vibrancy idle, and lets it back up again. The question is, do we sit, or walk? There is no answer.

We are here to guide. We are here to oblige. We are here to shake the fence upon which the world sits. There is a lamp-post near where we all live – and it's here we see in the darkness. It is not unknown to see someone standing under it at night.

Changing direction, we rattle in to the dazed and the berated. – they suffer, so they win. We climb the hill to the next stop. It is morning here, and the sun is out. We clamber forward, and in an instant, are being looked after. This much consoles.

Going for the tin, never more than in haste. I believe in further strides, but much is amass with the diamond. But what should we do, with an open heart and an open soul – should we close them up? Let suffering do its thing.

There is a dimension to things that alleviates as it dispenses. And here we find solace, and here our wounds are clean. We must not pour density into any wound. Only to say – this much is precluded.

Also, we shouldn't intend suffering (to self or others - or other living beings), but rather should harvest suffering as it natural arises. This much is fine.

A note here on ethics. We are talking about the transformation of suffering. In doing so, it is important that we act in accordance with a system of principles or precepts that are governed by a belief system we share. It doesn't really matter which one. It could be Christian, Buddhist, Aristotelean, an ethic of what we eat such as being vegetarian or vegan. It could be the philosophy of Confucious. Whatever system you subscribe to, ethics are essential to living the life of a suffering practitioner, if we call it this. It can also be your own ethical philosophy, however it may form.

And then, like a trail through the undergrowth, we watch and do not succumb. We tarry for the hills, but what does that give us, except the exorbitance of the style of it. Come now we mark the while in forever. Be the time it takes. We will catch a hold.

Aficionados of taste and belief. We encounter nothing short of everything here. There is a transformation of all sorts that goes on. The fire inside diminishes, but is replaced by the well and the ochre. There comes a time for allaying fears.

Come and be the sense we have to ride again.
Come and be what the journey has already told
us. There is a name for this in streaks of all out
abandon. Do not feather the plaster, it sticks to
what is worn. I know of nothing else like this. It will
be there.


Forming an opinion, but one that is not required to
be requitted. Forming something in the way of it.
Forming a force to be achieved. Forming
something more than we can give to the grass.
We are never circumspect, only in the mountains.


We are often divisive, but only when things are
brought to a head. We transplant the
rhododendrons to see if they will be still. There is
a sense we have that the fault is in the lines –
lines is the sand, as it presented by the sun.



An issue with the ease of it. We come, and then
stay, and then incite but not ignite. There is a
passion amongst the rocks. A passion that never
tarries, but is always aloft. We sometimes see
ourselves in the gust of it – and here we are
reminded.


Fixing what we need, and only on that basis.
There is a dimension to outgrow, and out parry the
winding of sticks through summer air. There is

something we must only be able to do once a day – and what is that? We will embark.

A bitterness that doesn't last. A cordial introduction. We simmer, as we must, but nothing more. We are of the ages – to who knows where. There is a likeness to the stars that the heavens repeat. And then as in one of each of the cases, we breathe.

And then, like the fibre in a meal set, we honour our delight with the rest of life. Come now, for the vision of the ineffable we encounter – we never see the way in and out of it. There is a motion here, that treads unto the day unto the night.

A mistaken reddish hue, of a type we cannot belong to. I trudge, but only when there is time. I see the marble, and know it to be a thing of beauty. I harbour nothing out of sight. There is here something we cannot explain. But we must continue.

Forging new life. We come once more to the epitome of hovering. It is here we have as the rice and the dish, something of the culinary, but not all. It is to the engaging of the piece we flourish, and let see the distance. There will be a difference.

## And for a Moment Everything Seemed Fine

Four score and ten – we little by little move in a definite arc. There is not much left to give, but what there is can be salvaged as such. A tendency to go with it. A flight in the morning that doesn't let up. There is something we cannot explain.


Just to be, to be in action, and in the sway. To be, with venom and denouncing. To be, with a heart of deliverance. To be without even thinking. Just to be. With hardly a need on the ground, we hop, and hop to it. And then? Oh yes, indeed.


A fortune in the wind. It tethers a river of five. And then, incredulous, incredulous we bend. Not for the sport, but for the sheer translucency of the light. We echo, but for what? We time ourselves, but from when? The danger is in the wood.


A near perfect resolution – chimed as it had from mysteries incarnate. We sense the outlying motion of the sky to be a renegade retrograde one, without the need to fall. Come and be the task we bare, one that labours with strength to encumber.


Hovering, like a new wave, like tinsel, like a splash, like any-which-way, like there, like now, like the tail of it. I send the spiral spinning. And here, where the misanthrope guides, but guides only, we message the hold for another look.

The is never a force strong enough to silence the reams that fate has at its disposal. There comes a bristle in the catch, and a simplicity in the weave. I know of something that will excite, above all measure. What is it? You will see.

And now – time is a harvester, harvester of souls. There is my excitation. Please do not be offended – we cause to erupt. And here, like a spent force, we love, and admire, and see the downfall of empires, mighty and renowned. We will switch.

The night is gravy, so says the oracle. And there with winged teeth, an action that bares nothing, nothing but all. We test the limits of what can and can't be done. But that is the limit of the turn and the web. Do not find the grass to show. It will pass.

Weathering, and away. A sort of tart, that is only served once a year. A willingness to collapse. And then, like a burning from the stare, new life, and the visage of the old. I plan with this composure to enable the wings to move us, through the air.

A gnashing of teeth – one that doesn't salt the jar. And then, in time to a forgotten dance, we move in the way of the wisp. 'Wisp to you good sir'. 'Wisp to you madam'. I appraise. And then notice the mystery of it all.

Suffering – we notice nothing more, nothing less.
It is here for us to stop its assails. We must revel
in the good it does us after we encounter it. Our
lives improve, if we take suffering in the right way.
And that we cannot avoid – it is evolutionary.


Much to say at least – much to talk about. Much to
render through and away. We catch the
perpendicular, and somersault through the hoops.
And jingle around the corner, like a bear that
cannot be tamed. We listen only because we can.


Forests, and lakes, and all that resides in beauty
and the decisive. We marshal our delays, to be in
time for the prevalence of the venture. And here,
where the troop does not disband, a flailing and a
giving ground. I hope the resting here is solid.


Whatever that is like the chain, we break.
Whatever that is like the chain we give our most
ardent composure to the crew. And then like a
magnificence in according, we dazzle our way up
the stairs, through the gate, and up towards, and
beyond.


We are walking slower than we ever have. But this
much does not turn us. We quicken our step, and
we feel the heart go, and the muscles. There is

never a loose step. It is a precession of the soul (sole). We will find a way.

Fasting before the fight, we love the motion in-between the shore and the sea. Do not blemish the record – or do so, and then run the mile in return backwards. There is nothing new about the pose. It comes with a flash and a drum.

Do not distribute the calm. Have as an anchor the choice of it, and be there when the mission enjoys. I will halve the marrow, and have as its source the winding of bitter tears. I have heard the noise coming from rooms. It will desist.

Suffering in the vociferous – we arch our backs, and know that in time, we will have what we need. There is license enough to send the missive to the caretaker for support. It wrenches and searches, and plays back on harbours entrenched.

Winding through – up and down. We catch a glimpse of the roadside on our way. It is a milestone – not long to go now. We shimmy, right and left, and in-between. And here, where the fibre of life is at its apex, here, we fumble through the hills.

Not knowing which way to go – we hear the confabulation at a pinch. And like a box of tissues in the night, we find ourselves, deep within. There is a part of us that boils down to the ground, and a part that smarts and giggles to the placement.

A scissor kick, one that is not of this world. We laugh and hurry, and find ourselves ready, ready for the march of ages. It is here we find depth, and here we sing a song, a new song, one that beleaguers only those who hear it.

Running around the garden – there are petals on the grass there, and raiments to be seen. I have as the merry way those who will come, and those not. But in the chase of it, a charm – one that determines the vacuity of the space.

Masculine, and renowned. Dealing in the whole of it. Never once for the fashion of it. We stand, and stand again. We write our lives in unison. But it is here where the consideration erupts. We hang on, but what do we taste? We will know.

Fortune, and waste. We gather, but for what intrigue? We harp, but for what endeavour? There are mysteries here in the weave. We own the bench, but have not sought the consort. There is a paradigm not missing. We arch, and that is the fray.

A tip-toe through the invigoration of a soul at night.
I am finished with the basting. I have not the
stomach for it. I lunge at myself in the mirror.
There are more things here than a rowdy
dissemination. I will hunt the series in two.


Up and across. Hardship, and improvement. This
is the score to settle, and we will settle it. It is the
heightening of consciousness that brings us there.
It commands a grand view of what your life is
going to be like. Give in to it.


A faulty bridge. One that sets the street ablaze.
This is the tempest. This is the sight. This is all
that should be, and all that ever was. We come to
be closer to the heart. We come to be closer to the
neckless of the touch. Here and always.


An imagination – strength and courage. We leave
in the trail of our lives much that has as its goad
the treacle of consideration. There is a likeness to
the hub. But what brings forth the daily rind – such
that impediments do not arise?


There is life here. But what of the sound, the
sound of the round? We argue in keepsakes and
in spires. There can be no more than this. There
can only be what we choose to transfigure. And
here a laze to mend the out-take.

A lasting solace. One that harbours joy as it does the night. I am here, where journeymen whisper. I am here where the solstice brings. Do not alleviate the charm, it is here for good. Do not linger in the wood. Simply go.


A far away capacity. We yoke ourselves to the task. But there is a sweetness, like now. There is a new day every day. There is here a sense of single mindedness that worries deep, but releases. I am of the opinion of hope. I am of the way of it.


And then, we encounter our first sufferings of the day. We must keep in mind the transformation that occurs. If we can do that, we are home. The suffering can't touch us then. It is as if it has become frozen – and cannot affect us. This is it.


A great rhythm moves the water and the sand. It is here where we can never faint or pass out. There is too much to do, too much to belong to. We have as the receptacle a prolonged encasement. It is as if we were no longer there.


A further glance is all we need. A further enchantment to wisp us along to the place of ease. I engender the victory of yore, and have as a template the seeming clarity of a touch. We do not hinder the chance of redolent charm.

What is left of this? What is left of the victory and the motioning? There is now a test of strength. We augur the will to be polished. We never reprimand the tile, nor the sink. There is a time for all this in the way. Do not descend – we await.

A causing glance, we inhibit no further. I will guide you here – guide you to that place behind the forest door. What doesn't please us will remain aloof. What doesn't cause the air to constrict is something fine. There is now a force of nature.

The nearness, and the furthest. The wanting, and the crash. We absolve, and then capitulate to the hearsay. Do not rejuvenate the dawn, it is here to stay. We gather ourselves for the circumference. It is here new life is born.

A delivery here. We notice the sign of it is not adhered. But that shouldn't bother the wheel burrow. It is a mixture of this to that, up to down. There is something in the wind. It is the sea. It is the radiant, and the turnbuckle. We will be still.

We encounter suffering every day. Why not have our revenge, and turn the tide a little, by making suffering pay a price. And that price is to give us the means to improve our lives, one bit of suffering at a time. Brilliant.

There is now a place – a place we have made ourselves – a place we can go to whenever we want. It is here the time it takes is a passage. It is here, that the misanthrope has the dimension to faulter, and begin again.

We hush, and beyond this motion, is the register of finality, finality as it stands. In the layout, there is nothing like this. In the temperance of scathing bite, we will travel again to the centre, and cause the rite to fall and rise once more.

A belief in things to come. What more is that? What more is the sound of the string through the air? I follow you, without compunction. But you are the need, as I am the tether. We will gather rightly – and sing for the rest of it. Here we will be.

A commiseration. You have come too late. But wait – this is the travail and the score. We catch the dire and the weak in strengths of odd application. Do not range, we are at that site that should only be reticent by the ancient and the bored. Yes.

We test everything for what it is worth. And then, like the vanquished and the tried, we elongate to see what is what. A new morsel, one that doesn't flinch. A new insight – one we wish to share. This is the space and the carving. We will not relent.

Folding, and leaving. Being what cannot be bought. Being the sense and the nonsense. Being what cares. I have touched the basin before now. It is something not for me to see. I love, but am postponed. I catch sight, but only in the winter.

One more plank gone from suffering's arsenal. We are winning this war. It will come at us, stronger than ever. But we will not back down. Suffering is ours for the taking. Before long, complete and utter victory – imagine that.

Very still. Like a range in the cumbersome. Like a feather in the mill. Like a short sharp soliloquy. One that doesn't decry the world. We admonish the very sound of it. This much is not to stand. This much is only to diminish.

A treasure to perceive. A look of alabaster, and thought to care. We rotate the pieces in line with the columns. What is left, I hear you say? Nothing in serviceable amounts. We have as an element the writing on the square. There there.

A missing piece, a piece that ruptures into finality. We are the loss, and not the reason. But reason has us, like so much smog. We counter, and then remiss. We hold on, but not for the cry. There is time to be at the loggerhead.

Aforementioned titles, awaiting the need of suns. We augment through whistle stop tours, and conventional attires. We deliver on the trace. But a far cry from the top. There is a working of the present that holds us. And yes, like a gambler at high noon.

A light post – standing, observing, having as a reminder. Nothing inhibits like the show. Nothing feels its way to the start, as much as this. There is a cumbersome reward nestled in. Do not believe the water, it comes to us together.

A feeling like the sands of it. The next mix is often a good one. I hear it said, and then transmute. I never stagger, only to show how it is done. And then, like a rice-cake eaten with vigour, we catch sight of the daylight, and have our share.

What is suffering? Why does it come? Why is it here? What sense does it make? Its truth is that it can be transformed. It is now on the back foot. Imagine, after a year of suffering, we can visualise what we need or want, and manifestation occurs.

Cornering in. We catch sight of all that is precious to us. And here, where we have laboured so long, a chance to breathe again. There is a temptation to shout, but yet not be inhibited. There sings the nightingale, resplendent.


I will ask you a question. 'What is made for laughter, but catches only tears?' I will leave that one with you. And then, an embarking, one that never stops. I am one to listen closely, only because it is rare. There is a nightly scribe – we will fuse.


A sea of fits and spits. We counter our point through the trembling of the majority. There is a point of reference that has now been engaged. And here, where the minutest commonplace stays still, we own the fore-shore, and commiserate.


Foregone and alive. At most, the seeds to carry. I will angle the barter where it never was. And now, the ardent and the frost. The cold, and the sequel. What can no longer divide is shown its course. We are want to scramble, and we do.


Etching closer – like never before. We hold our task, and bundle the cray, and see the distance like it was here. There is a time for us. It comes now. We are the leaning, and the pinafore. We hold on, just despite.


A piece of the sublime. We gather like hearts; we feel the commonplace like ranges. We open up the discussion, and give back what has been unruly. I invest myself in the pleasure of it. There is no smirk above the grade. We will observe.


We suffer – but for what purpose? For this purpose of transformation. As a suffering practitioner for many years, I have channelled my suffering into my writing, to great success. Every bit of suffering I encounter gets transformed.


Marginalised, and repudiated. A swinging that longs. A piece of jetsam that holds the key. And now, all we need do, is visualise what takes us. And in that grasp, we are found again. In that grasp – we encounter all that suffices.


A ready pall, one that says, I am sure. We have as the rest of life a litany of the foregoing. We clasp, and then go through. We worship, and have the sound of the tempest engage us like a busy-ness to behold. Never once but thrice.


A languishing that doesn't last. A hope that we have that things will turn out. A new fashion in the weave. Cosmopolitan and intriguing. Raining like the window that looks out onto the street. We must not stop. For anything, or anyone.


Bearing in mind – what can be done once can be done a thousand times. And here, where we loll about for the test of it, we come in vast signature array. It is like we never were. It is now we speak to the forge to prepare our armour.


There, there in the distance. I see you there. I see you. I am one to joust with folly. I have as the introduction all that I can bring. Inching forward, I give the cast a thousand breezes, one for each day, between now and then.


There is a fashion to uphold. There is a stake to claim. There is a noise that does not listen. There is all this and more. I do not insist, but only whisper. There is light beyond the fence line. We do not contribute, anything at all. This much is done.


I have heard, that suffering is surmountable. I have heard that it can be surpassed. It is a phenomenon that never rests, but we can stop it, we have the tools. Think about how much suffering human beings have gone through throughout the centuries. We have simply adapted. When we encounter suffering, it just provides us with the means towards improvement.


Having the right, being able, and singing. Being in the middle of all that is, and shouting for it. Being the constant in a turning world. Being over-abundant, but enjoying the cast. I hope you enjoy the show.

And for a Moment Everything Seemed Fine

A ferocity, and then being resplendent. A future thoroughfare that has as its endeavour all that time will give. I am wanting to say more, but am trickled into recalcitrant threads. But here it is, in all its renown. Let us now proceed.

There is a feeling that the centuries cannot abide. There is a testing that does not harbour, nor release at any juncture. I hear the salience of the tributaries coming down to this. I will pull up in time, and then rush through the arc of it.

I have as a life all the trials of the wind. Everyone. But when we encounter the freight from the heights to the depths, here a massaging of lifelines co-mingle, and never rear for a single moment. I have as the tools the sequin mass. I will use them, today.

A sense of calm – what is it for? What lies in untold distances. What is the house on the hill for? I quickly transpose the vengeance post, the ground will never hear it. I lounge, but for what applause? I sink, but there is nothing new in that.

A kaleidoscopic deportment, one that rings in April blue. I sense a furthering, to the tune of the nomenclature. Witness this – there is a road in the hills – one that goes through, around and beyond.

We witness vast feats – feats of strength above all.

We sublimate what we encounter, and let our lives slowly but surely get better. Our suffering, for a time gets better, and then increases again, depending upon what we want. That is all suffering is for. For the transformation of our lives.

There is something we have not seen. It is here, here in the radish sale. I give the solace we find a new home, and have what is naught in transcendence, reap higher echelons, ones that do not curtail nor invite. This is what we say.

A nice time to bite. A time like no other. We rinse our mouths, but only because the taste of life lingers. I know of no other charm, nor matter of fact resorting, than this – purity as it is. Do you climb steeply, and then liken the way to the antechamber?

Following the lead, and seeing it through. Much is said of the compass and the stall. Much that we should only consider in transit and without rush. I liken the hay to the wire, and all that scoops the cellophane into things. Be brief – we are told.

A new way of baring. A sort of accompaniment. Lists of the steering. We envelope the crowd, in this time frame and the next. What have we felt, but all? What have known, but much? There is a skirting board that unties – we will mesh.


We come crashing, and gnashing, and all that is temperate. I shine on the stage, but only because you are there too. I long for the blast of highlights, and desires in one. There can only be a misnomer where we walk. This much reverberates.


What is it we have found? What is it we have seen? We trudge, but for the height. We live in dreams of commitment. Be a harrowing that drowns the rest out. There is neither the here nor the now. These things live as brothers and sisters of the yore.


What would life be like without suffering? What would our lives be like? Suffering would still be there, but we wouldn't feel it. And we would still be there. It is hard to think of – a life without suffering. But who knows? A reality maybe.

We cause the slumber to dream. This encases us in heart. We stand firm, like a distant ratification. I know of no other way. There are languishments that can never curtail. I hear the rummaging, and know that the climb is here.


I sense a movement in place. One that swings and arches, and has as a refurbishment all the while.

The coach draws near. We will catch it to where we want to go. And in this, a champion of stars glisten. One beside the next.


And now we repeat the scale of it. There is a rising and a judging, and all that life has to commit to. We will never know the boundaries in the without. We approve of the acceptance, but will it last? There can be nothing more.


Finding a new lease of the living. I cannot evoke more here than elsewhere. There is a touch that heals, there is a wound that cannot spread. There is a rainbow in earshot, and here we follow ourselves through dark and grey.


A worn and torn exuberance. What is the surmise? What toils? What catches the rapidity? We linger, but only in salt. I slow, and then remember my allotment. This is like the rest. And with this we detail what is nearing.


A reverberation, one that harks together through the sound. There is a mesmerising at work. We will listen. There are chimes that work in spades, and leanings that do not otherwise. We harvest to metal, and see it cross, to be capable.


There is a lot to live through. And in this our suffering has a lot to answer for. We could permit ourselves a glimpse of life without suffering – what would it be like? There is a mystery here only we can tame. A life without suffering. Goose bumps.


There is a road here – a road no one has travelled on yet. And then like a simple thing, made even simpler, we walk down this road – but what do we find? Our pace is steady, the road has many undulations. We will find a place to sleep.


Having something like-minded, and having it come with us. It is like we never parted. And then, like a static in the wind, we embark, and know all to be well. I feel the gale – but to what effect? There is a liberality to it. And here we find.


Coming closer now, we find our voice. We can't say that is about time, but we can now envisage. Envisage what? Life – our life together on this journey. We see ourselves in vast array. Causing nothing to be otherwise.


There is a magnetism about the fluidity of it. We launch, and have as the stall all that partakes of it. There is no time to better ourselves further. What is done is done. We are left to count clocks, and do so in the rain. We will lavish.


A near take on an old road. I have as the august and the rail much to be intrigued by. There is a simplicity of desires that rides the coach of souls. It wrinkles freely, and denotes all who will come. This much is told in the plan of things.


A question of halves. A burning that leaves its mark. I will not have the round for all of the pittance renowned. Come and find the safeguard – it is of importance. And now we gather at the fjord. Only to hear the rhythm that is made. Yes, it is free.


What is suffering? It is a question that may never be answered. We may know on our death beds, but what we can tell now is limited. It comes, wreaks, and goes, followed by a sense of relief. We may never really know what it is.


Forests of silence. Not a living thing. An ocean can never be silent. What we listen to is the breeze of it. What we listen to is the sound of the cold. It has a sound, much like rain. Much like the storm. We are living, and here we are.


Hanging on, despite. Despite everything, and anything. Despite the cost, and the bow. Despite all that wagers in the district. I have as the merry seekers a glance at the time. There is a functioning that weaves in and out of doubt. There.

## And for a Moment Everything Seemed Fine

A forbearance that militates against the grain. What is here, will never be there. What is now, can never be then. We open our hearts, and give our trust in things a push. And like something out of the aquarium, we revisit ourselves anew.

There is a chance to be seen with fresh eyes, and heard with fresh ears. And then like the tightrope, we balance, and head to the spring for a recovery. This is all that is to it. This is all we must do. I settle, and embark again.

Mischievous, and with a solemnity to tag. We still the motion and the semblance. We drive the closeness and the rapidity. There is nothing more elusive than this. I try all the curtailments, and find the one. And here like a renegade we sing.

Having a shout – never more knowing what is in favour. We laugh, and say our graces. We let be, and know the way home. There is a mine as deep as the guest. We love, and spill, and fire, and light, and give all that can be given.

There is more to life than this. Our suffering keeps us chained. Chained to the wheel. But now we can use it to better our lives – to furnish our lives with new and endearing things, states of mind, points of pleasure.

A waterfall – one we know, and cannot dispel.
Here we love what we are, and know that the right
is left, and all that partakes is an open field – an
open field of readiness. What is the motion of the
world to us? We give our labouring new life.


A crescent moon – what do we see in it? All that is
curious – curious as the light that shines. We are
incensed at the chosen mission, and all that
comes to the mighty. I have a plan, one that does
not entice, nor vanquish the uneven.


Stumbling through the dark – we find a way
forward. It is here we feel most alive – with hairs
bristling, and the cumbersome for the naught. I
have guessed at speed, and know the lancing of
the test is all that we need to do.


Temptations to demise – we are the brittle and yet
the strong. We gather rose petals for the
ceremony. We are what has come, and never left.
When we do leave, it is for the air we breathe and
the somnolent amongst us.


Deliberately letting the water in. Never reminiscing
– always holding on. We love it when things come
together. And in that there is an embrace. I have
as the motion, a silent respect. I have as the line a
marker – a marker of all that will be.

Occurring at the same time, but not being deficient. There are torches for the darkness. There are things that bloom in the day. I have as a solidity all that cannot be vanquished. Dust and clovers, and the temporality of it.


We speak, but not of this world. We co-operate, but only to see the night. There is here something we have not known of. We will learn to admonish, and have as the joy a third-party, one that dances on the trail, only to disappear through.


A magic – this is our experience with suffering. Imagine we can transform our suffering, which we can. There is now a new place for suffering. With our heightening of consciousness, we can achieve what we want – and inevitably finish suffering.


A very pleasurable experience. We laugh, and test ourselves, and have as fate all the muses can bear. There comes to the sight of it, a new turn of phrase. Here, where we are now, is a soft place – gone are the railings.


A sentimental cry. We love to see what you are doing now. And then, like a hardship felt and then forgotten, we linger, and decide on which way to turn. There embarks a new quest, one that lives in ancient memory. This is the toast.

A mismatch of clothes – but what of it? We angle like sight, and have as the darling to encounter nothing short of the intrepid. Love life. It comes for the sport. It never encounters the drum. And then, like a pair of doves, sanctuary and release.


Misguided understandings. A weathering that heals. What we had never thought, what we had never seen. I ask this of you – that in my company you should be kind. That in my company you shall prevail. Can I ask that?


I endeavour to succumb. I endeavour to be heard. I fear, but only in equal measure. I love, but only so that we both can live. Within the partisan of the creed, we have something of the outdoors to reconcile. Do not be long in shouting.


Why suffering? Why in our world? It could have been a lack of suffering. But it is here – so we must act. We have the formula for the transformation – but a good deal of awareness is also required. With that, our lives become buoyant.


The giant within. The giant to guard. We have what it takes. And then like a manoeuvre at half pace, we come. We are not left here to wonder, nor talk in tones of gold. We are here to work, and then to wander, and then chisel away.

## And for a Moment Everything Seemed Fine

I ask a favour of the ocean - sweep me out as far as you can, but then let me swim back in. Allow me do this. Then I am thankful, and can rest. It is like the bar has been raised, and the noise it makes has further encased itself in blue.

Dusting off the weather, we catch ourselves in the wind again. But that is what it is for, to be tested. And then, like a sail unfurled, we witness a new form of heart. It is here we stay, and here we fight, and here we walk for the tundra.

Gorgeous to the eye, swept up by the feet – beleaguered in enhancement. Always casting the time. We halt, and derive, and then move forward, before halting again. This is the way of it, and as it should be. Reticence comes, to be turned.

Just in time. Just because. I limit what comes before me so as not to overwhelm. I touch on silk, only because of the rain. There is a sulking, but then a joy. I have as the sunlight a time for missing. There, and there abouts. We will swing.

Coming up for air, our speed is on par. We set foot, but only because we can. There is something deep within – something we can't explain. I will try and explain it – before I forget – it is gone. A pile of bric-a-brac on the side of the road.

There comes a chance at redemption – we must take it. But what forms does it take? What sounds does it make? What could it possibly mean? There is a breath to it – we can hear it. There is something now we should do – fall in line, and then release.


Suffering – it is hard to define – such is its breadth and scope. Maybe pain, maybe hardship, maybe discomfort, maybe all of that. But we know when we encounter it, and when we get used to it, seeing past transformations around us.


A gain, a sweepstake – a mettle in amongst it. We thrive, only to let the passage way clear. We open the gates, and the flood comes. We chose life over the water. And before we can even begin again, we are transposed like a river through rust.


What is the time for? Does it measure? Is it covered in memories? Does it harbour the wind, and all that blows? Is this what we should say of it – much sense. We will always remember what has come – dearest and brightest.


A place for the striving, and to heal. A place for the reticent, and the recalcitrant. We are left with nothing out of the ordinary, but only this – an address we dreamed of only the night before. We now see it clearly, and will travel.

And for a Moment Everything Seemed Fine

There comes a time for the widow to take hold of life, and send to the outer reaches all that pretends to be safety. There is a tremendous delay, one that weeps tears of sugar and nourishment. See the tenacity of syrup, see it as it shines.

A block of wood. The sculptor. All that will pass as shape. We intuit the surrounds, and give as the recondite a new fashioning. There is a much-needed surmise, one that arcs at the margins. We will come for the laughter, and stay for the shade.

Touching the scar, we find ourselves remembering how it happened. There is a shape to this abandon, one that seeks in covers born of the guild. I will not let the fire go out. I will not underlie what is to come. There is time enough.

What is it to suffer, anyway? We feel suffering – it has a bodily aspect. We have an aversion to it, that is clear. It incites pain, both in the body and the emotions. We can now situate it, and use it for our purposes. Suffering – multifaceted.

A dream – but a dream of what? We have as our incentive the arranging of chairs at the end of the night. But this cannot be the only thing. There is a muse that governs this sort of beautification. We argue, but only for the time remaining.


A hark, and then a hallow. Are you there, my friend? I believe him to be. There is no chase like this one. There is now a bottle of vinegar to store. It is here amongst the mangroves, here is the perfect place. Sing, and be sought.


A restful night, and a day of the adventure. Quite the recipe. We will gather our treasures, and see them soar. What is left unto the light of the moon. What causes our grief is now here today. There seems a natural place for things.


Getting closer – closer to what matters. And here, with sympathy, and a heavy heart, we know that time is a magnet, one that never flinches. We long, and have as the guest a piece of fabric – one that never un-weaves.


A festivity is struck, for those all encumbered. We look sparse, but feel great – all in one. The message is this – do not denounce this life, but rather manage it as a form of toil. This much makes sense. We come to breath, and that will find sequence.


After the play, we chatted – and here, we formed two of a rock. And in this motion, something to list.